新医科英语系列教材

AN ELEMENTARY COURSEBOOK
FOR MEDICAL ENGLISH

医学英语基础教程

总主编◎黄立鹤　吴　赟

主　编◎宋　缨

副主编◎刘　丽

编　者◎孙　丹　朱锡明

　　　　辛　燕　史其慧

　　　　万晓蒙

清华大学出版社

北　京

内 容 简 介

本教材共八章，内容涉及免疫系统、预防医学、慢性病、癌症、替代医疗（也称另类医疗）、营养、心理健康和医学道德。本教材在以英语语言教学为重心的基础上，帮助学生了解相关医学知识，并熟悉医学学科的语言特征和话语范式。每个章节设有课前阅读、课文、课文注解、词汇表、课后练习、语块知识点小讲座等环节，旨在提升学生用英语进行医学专业领域交流的技能和批判性思维能力。

本教材适合普通高校大学英语教学范畴中的专门用途英语课程教学，也可供广大英语爱好者自学使用。本教材配有优质音频资源，学生可直接扫码听音。

图书在版编目（CIP）数据

医学英语基础教程 / 黄立鹤，吴赟总主编；宋缨主编. — 北京：清华大学出版社，2023.8
新医科英语系列教材
ISBN 978-7-302-64365-4

Ⅰ. ①医…　Ⅱ. ①黄…　②吴…　③宋…　Ⅲ. ①医学－英语－教材　Ⅳ. ①R

中国国家版本馆 CIP 数据核字（2023）第 149804 号

责任编辑：白周兵
封面设计：张伯阳
责任校对：王凤芝
责任印制：沈　露

出版发行：清华大学出版社
　　　　网　　　址：http://www.tup.com.cn, http://www.wqbook.com
　　　　地　　　址：北京清华大学学研大厦 A 座　　　　　　邮　　编：100084
　　　　社 总 机：010-83470000　　　　　　　　　　　　邮　　购：010-62786544
　　　　投稿与读者服务：010-62776969, c-service@tup.tsinghua.edu.cn
　　　　质量反馈：010-62772015, zhiliang@tup.tsinghua.edu.cn
印 装 者：三河市天利华印刷装订有限公司
经　　销：全国新华书店
开　　本：185mm×260mm　　　　　印　　张：16.75　　　　字　　数：340 千字
版　　次：2023 年 8 月第 1 版　　　　　　　　　　　　印　　次：2023 年 8 月第 1 次印刷
定　　价：69.00 元

产品编号：097838-01

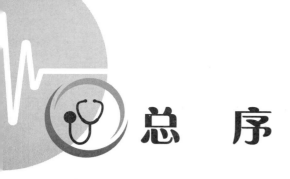

总　序

　　中华人民共和国成立以来，特别是改革开放以来，我国健康领域的改革发展取得了显著成就；近 10 年来，健康中国战略全面实施，人民健康得到全方位保障，我国走出了一条中国特色卫生健康事业改革发展之路。医学教育是卫生健康事业发展的重要基石，党的十八大以来，我国把人民健康放在优先发展的战略地位，医学教育蓬勃发展，高素质医学人才脱颖而出。面对实施健康中国战略的新任务、世界医学发展的新要求，我国仍需把医学教育摆在教育和卫生健康事业优先发展的地位。

　　随着我国持续推进卫生健康国际交流合作、深入参与全球卫生治理，健康医疗领域人员跨国界、跨地区流动已是大势所趋，国际化能力培养在我国医学教育发展中愈加受到重视。《国务院办公厅关于加快医学教育创新发展的指导意见》（国办发〔2020〕34 号）（下称《指导意见》）明确指出，要"培养具有国际视野的高层次拔尖创新医学人才"。 2020 年 6 月，教育部临床医学专业认证工作委员会以"无条件通过"的结果正式获得世界医学教育联合会（WFME）医学教育认证机构认定，这标志着我国医学教育标准和认证体系实现国际实质等效，医学教育认证质量得到了国际认可。毫无疑问，提升健康医学领域人才的国际化视野和能力是落实我国"新医科"教育理念的重要方面。

　　为进一步落实"新医科"教育中的国际化能力培养，提升健康医学专业学生的英语应用能力，我们深度参与了"新医科英语系列教材"的编撰工作，主要承担《医学英语基础教程》《医学英语阅读教程》《医学英语写作教程》《医学人文英语教程》《临床医学英语教程》《中医药英语实用教程》等教材的编写。本套教材围绕与健康医学相关的众多议题，落实加快以疾病治疗为中心向以健康促进为中心的转变，体现"大健康"理念，覆盖基础医学、临床医学、中医药、医学技术、公共卫生、医学人文、医学史、医学哲学等各类题材，涉及健康医学领域的核心范畴、前沿技术、行业标准、历史文化、健康治理等内容。体裁丰富多样，包含说明文、议论文、记叙文、应用文及人物访谈等。教材构思新颖，如把语块教学理念融入基础语言教学，设置真实医学临床实践和研究场景的英语教学，凸显基于医学英语任务的思辨创新能力培养，启发不同健康医学活动背后的跨文化思考，引导学生利用网络信息平台查找专业信息，介绍医工、医理、医文等学科交叉融合的前沿内容等。练习形式有趣、内涵丰富，要求学生对健康医学领域的实际问题进行创新性解决，从而实现英语语言能力和医药卫生专业视野的双向拓展。

全面推进课程思政建设是落实立德树人根本任务的战略举措。《指导意见》明确指出，要"强化医学生职业素养教育，加强医学伦理、科研诚信教育，发挥课程思政作用"，从而培养仁心仁术的医学人才。在编写中，我们始终牢记英语教学的育人功能，融入中国立场、价值伦理、职业素养等内容，潜移默化地引导学生逐步树立良好医德。我们努力平衡语言难度、学术深度、人文温度、历史厚度，在医学科学与语言人文中寻找结合点，力图打造一套既能体现医学人文思想，又兼具国际视野和家国情怀的高水平医学英语教材。

本套教材参照教育部《大学英语教学指南（2020版）》的课程设置要求，兼顾专门用途英语和通用英语；同时，参考《高等职业教育专科英语课程标准（2021年版）》，兼顾英语课程结构中的基础模块和拓展模块。因此，本套教材呈现一定的难度进阶，既可以作为应用型本科或高职高专医药卫生类专业的英语教材，也可作为普通高校本科阶段大学英语教学中的医学专门用途英语教材，个别教材甚至可用于英语类专业课堂教学或课后阅读材料使用；同时，它在一定程度上还适合愿意学习国际健康医学相关内容的社会人士，可满足临床医学、护理、药学、医学技术、卫生管理等方向的英语学习需要。

本套教材由同济大学发起，联合北京大学（含医学部）、山东大学、陕西师范大学、扬州大学、黑龙江大学、曲阜师范大学、四川外国语大学、上海中医药大学（及附属龙华医院）、天津中医药大学、广西医科大学、济宁医学院、南京工业职业技术大学、山东医学高等专科学校等高校，邀请医学英语教学、健康话语研究等领域内经验丰富的专家、教师和医生充分研讨、共同编写而成。同济以医学建校，学校始于1907年德国医生埃里希·宝隆在中德两国政府和社会各界支持下创办的医学堂，走的是一条由医而工、再到综合的发展之路。学校虽于20世纪50年代在全国高校院系布局调整中将医学院整体迁至武汉，但同济人医学情结至深，历经百年沧桑后，在新世纪之初重建医学。近年来，同济医科勇闯创新发展之路，结合世界医学发展前沿、未来趋势及国家需求，加快向国际一流水准迈进。

我们衷心希望本套教材能够配合深化医学教育改革，协助推进"卓越医生教育培养计划 2.0"，帮助学习者实现英语语言能力与医药卫生专业视野的双向拓展，培养其在健康医学领域进行国际交流合作的能力，成为我国推进卫生健康国际交流合作、参与全球卫生治理的重要人才。

黄立鹤　吴赟

2023 年 6 月于上海同济园

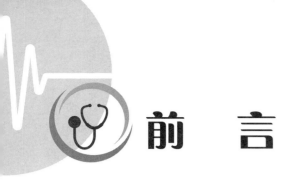

前　言

　　党的二十大报告提出要"深入实施科教兴国战略、人才强国战略、创新驱动发展战略"。在这一精神指引下，本教材编写组紧密对接国家发展"新医科"的重大决策，力争为高校公共英语教学开课列表中的专门用途英语模块提供一本新颖且实用的医学类教材。本教材旨在帮助学生在公共英语学习阶段强化英语语言基本技能的同时，了解医学学科的英语语言特征和话语范式，力争为高等院校医学专业英语的教学起到铺路石和对接的作用。

　　回顾近 20 多年，专门用途英语教学在国内各高等院校日益受到重视。虽已明确归属公共英语类开课范畴，但围绕该板块开展的教学似乎总与高等院校各院系开设的专业英语教学（也称全英语教学）存在着关系不清或职责混淆的现象，也由此引发各种激烈讨论。本教材试图从编写设计层面入手，来厘清这一"混乱"现象，以表达我们的理念——专门用途英语应侧重语言教学，而专业英语则应侧重行业知识传授。因此，本教材在强调语言基本技能全面发展的同时，多维度帮助学生熟悉医学领域的英语语言特征和规律。

　　本教材具有以下特色：

1. 坚定正确价值立场，服务课程思政建设

　　教材是育人的重要载体，直接关系人才培养方向和质量。因此，本教材在编写过程中始终坚持正确的价值导向和坚实的中国立场。例如，在章节选题方面，为呼应落实党的二十大报告提出的深入推进"健康中国"建设这一理念，我们设计了"替代医学"等特色章节，弘扬中国优秀传统文化，介绍中医药传承创新发展，以增强学生的文化自信。"预防医学""慢性病"等章节的编写，也直接对应"健康中国"建设中关于"坚持预防为主，加强重大慢性病健康管理；创新医防协同、医防融合机制"等任务。

2. 秉承专门用途英语使命，提升核心语言能力

　　本教材紧扣专门用途英语的特点，其编写以专业需求为驱动，以语言教学（language-based）为重心。首先，转变课程定位，即从通用英语转向专门用途英语，是确保教学取得成功的重要手段之一。教材编写只有紧密结合和充分考虑各专业院系对学生专业英语能力的需求，才能使公共英语从教材设计到教学手段更好地为特定领域的专业英语教学服务。其次，专门用途英语课程的教学目标不同于专业英语课程。前者是公共英语类课程，以语言教学为重心，重在把握学科中的语言使用规律和专业表达；而后者是各院系开设的专业课程，侧重内容（content-based）的专业知识教学，旨在通过英语这一语言载体来传授某个专门领域的学科知识。

作为一本专门学术英语教材，本教材的首要目标并非传授医学领域的学科知识，而是培养学生从词汇、句法、语篇等层面对医学专业文体进行辨析和归纳的能力，帮助学生了解医学学科的话语传统和规约，从而提高学生用英语在医学学科领域进行交流的能力。因此，本教材从章节选题到练习设计，都围绕上述两点展开。例如，我们在每一章都精心整理了与主题相关的常见医学词汇的构词元素，以帮助学生举一反三，轻松扩大医学词汇量；还特别编写了"特色两栖词汇表"，描述同一词汇在通用英语和医学英语中的不同含义，增强学生的识别意识和正确运用词汇的能力。练习设计遵循由浅入深、循序渐进的原则，引导学生在问题情境中进行思考。

3. 融入语块教学理念，创新语言学习方法

本教材将语块教学理念和专门用途英语教学进行融合。近些年，随着语料库语言学的发展，语块在外语教学与研究中越来越受到国内同行的重视，但基于语块理论的教材（chunks-based coursebook）不仅在通用英语教学中很少见，在专门用途英语教学中也可谓凤毛麟角。此外，专门用途英语课程是与各院系的专业英语最紧密对接的"排头兵"公共英语类课程，理应承担起其特有的重任，帮助学生提高在专业领域流利地用英语进行听、说、读、写、译的能力。基于上述考虑，本教材尝试增强学生对语块学习的意识，引导学生在学习新单词的同时，注重对已学单词的搭配进行探索。具体手段包括：对各章课文中的语块直接用黑体标注；在提供传统单词表（word list）的同时，还提供语块词汇表（chunk list）；每章末开设语块知识小讲座，系统介绍语块的理念、语块学习的重要性、语块的分类，以及行之有效的语块学习方法等。

本教材全体编者谨记教材是学校铸魂育人的关键要素，在医学英语领域中始终坚持正确的政治方向和价值导向，以高度的使命感、责任感和紧迫感，努力把打造精品落实到每一段文字、每一幅插图、每一道习题。教材编写过程中，中国人民解放军海

军军医大学李平老师提出了宝贵建议，在此表示感谢。衷心希望这本公共英语教学领域的专门用途英语类教材能有助于学生提高对医学英语语言特征的敏感性、医学语篇分析和信息识别能力，最终帮助他们更自信和顺利地走进全英语教学课堂，胜任医学专业英语的学习任务。

限于水平，本教材中一定还存在不少瑕疵，欢迎同行和使用者不吝赐教，帮助我们在修订或再版时做得更好。

编者

2023 年 2 月

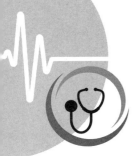

Contents

Chapter ① The Immune System

Chapter ② Preventive Medicine

Chapter ③ Chronic Illnesses

Chapter ④ Cancers

Chapter ⑤ Alternative Medicine

Chapter ⑥ Nutrition

Chapter ⑦ Mental Health

Chapter ⑧ Medical Ethics

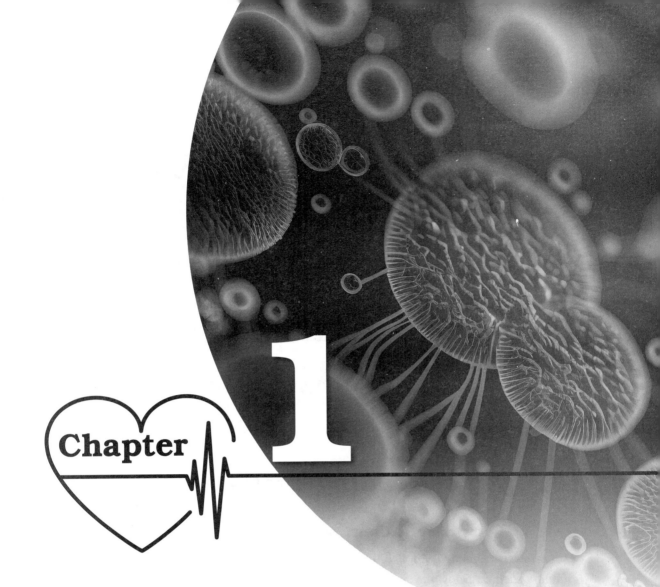

Chapter 1

The Immune System

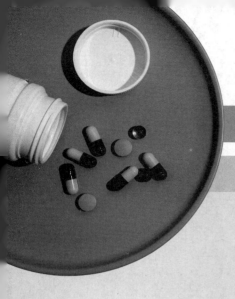

Chapter 1

The Immune System

Learning Objectives

- to master some basic skills to build medical words with affixes concerning the human immune system and to expand accurate usage of amphibious words in both general and medical contexts;

- to improve comprehensive linguistic abilities to discuss immunity;

- to increase awareness of the importance of the immune system and consciousness of boosting one's immunity.

Part 1　Pre-reading Tasks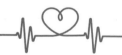

Task 1　Compare and Contrast

Directions: *In medical English, **amphibious words**, a term derived from amphibious animals such as frogs and toads that can live both on land and in water, have flexible meanings in both general contexts and medical contexts. Please consult your dictionaries, write down the Chinese equivalents of the amphibious words in the table below, and pay attention to their different meanings used as **general expressions (GE)** and **medical expressions (ME)** respectively. The first one is exemplified for you to follow.*

Amphibious Words	GE	ME
appendix	（书、文件等的）附录	阑尾
cold		
drop		
essential		
exposure		
host		
screen		

(Continued)

Amphibious Words	GE	ME
strain		
tissue		
ward		

Task 2 Read and Translate

Directions: Please read the following 10 pairs of sentences, and keep an eye on the 10 amphibious words you learned from the table in Task 1, which are interpreted differently as GE and ME. Translate the English sentences into Chinese.

1. For convenience, we have also provided a glossary in an <u>appendix</u>. (GE)

   _____

   _____

   With an acute inflammation of his <u>appendix</u>, he had to have it removed. (ME)

   _____

   _____

2. You'll catch a chill if you do not keep warm in <u>cold</u> weather. (GE)

   _____

   _____

   In winter or seasonal changes, the elderly or children are easy to suffer from a heavy <u>cold</u>. (ME)

   _____

   _____

3. It was stated that standards at the hospital were <u>dropping</u>. (GE)

   _____

   _____

   I have known the feeling of wearing contact lens without eye <u>drops</u>. (ME)

   _____

   _____

4. The <u>essential</u> character of the town has been destroyed by the new road. (GE)

_____

_____

The thesis is a study on early hearing impairment with <u>essential</u> hypertension. (ME)

_____

_____

5. All the candidates have been getting an enormous amount of <u>exposure</u> on television and in the press. (GE)

_____

_____

Travel increases the risk for <u>exposure</u> to measles virus and its further spread into susceptible populations if not vaccinated. (ME)

_____

_____

6. The college is playing <u>host</u> to a group of visiting Russian scientists. (GE)

_____

_____

When the eggs hatch, the larvae eat the living flesh of the <u>host</u> animal. (ME)

_____

_____

7. Government employees may be <u>screened</u> by the security services. (GE)

_____

_____

Men over 55 should be regularly <u>screened</u> for prostate cancer. (ME)

_____

_____

8. The dogs were <u>straining</u> at the leash, eager to get to the park. (GE)

_____

_____

The Delta <u>strain</u> is more transmissible, more adapted to humans and faster to replicate. (ME)

_____

_____

9. Under the circumstance of financial crisis, using less <u>tissue</u> means saving more money. (GE)

_____

_____

All the cells and <u>tissues</u> in the body benefit from the increased intake of oxygen. (ME)

_____

_____

10. He brought his arm up in a futile attempt to <u>ward</u> off the blow. (GE)

_____

_____

A toddler was admitted to the emergency <u>ward</u> with a wound in his chest. (ME)

_____

_____

Task 3 Lead-in Questions

Directions: Read the questions below and answer them in details.

1. Do you believe you are in good physical conditions? Why or why not?

_____

_____

2. What do you think of your lifestyle? Is it immunity-friendly?

   _____

   _____

3. What do you do in your everyday life to boost your natural defense system?

   _____

   _____

4. Do you think one's immunity system becomes weaker with aging? Will the conclusion you draw have some impact on your current lifestyle?

   _____

   _____

Part 2 Texts

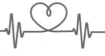

Text A

Understanding the ¹Immune System

1   The **immune system** is made up of cells and organs that protect your body from outside ²invaders such as ³bacteria, viruses, ⁴fungi, and ⁵parasites that can cause ⁶infection and disease. The immune system also **gets rid of** abnormal ⁷pre-cancerous cells and cancerous cells that are growing out of control. When it works correctly, it **fights off** infection and keeps you healthy. However, when the immune system is weak, ⁸germs and other abnormal cells in the body can more easily cause infections and diseases. Key organs and cells of the immune system are briefly discussed **as follows**.

2   The first line of defense against germs is your skin, the single largest organ of the body. It provides a physical barrier that keeps bacteria and viruses

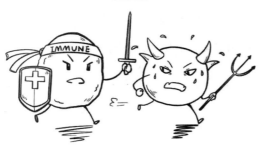

from entering the body. Viruses such as **HIV** cannot get through normal, healthy and unbroken skin. However, it can get into the body through unbroken [9]mucous [10]membranes.

3   The internal parts of your immune system **take care of** germs that do get inside the body. The **white blood cells** that defend the body from invaders and get rid of possibly dangerous abnormal cells, begin their lives in the **bone** [11]**marrow**. Once they leave the bone marrow, they travel to the [12]lymph organs, which serve as a **home base** for mature white blood cells. There, the white blood cells [13]await instruction to go out and fight infection.

4   Lymph organs are spread throughout the body and include the **lymph** [14]**nodes**, [15]thymus, [16]spleen, [17]appendix, etc. Lymph nodes are located in the neck, [18]armpits, [19]abdomen, and [20]groin. Each lymph node contains cells that are ready to fight invaders. The spleen is an important organ for a healthy immune system. It is about the size of a fist, and it is located in the upper left of the abdomen (also called "belly"). One of its key roles is to [21]filter blood and to identify and get rid of white blood cells that are **worn out**.

5   Some key cells of the immune system are [22]dendritic cells and [23]macrophages. Dendritic cells are found mostly in the skin and mucous membranes that protect the openings of the body (e.g. nose, mouth, and throat). These cells capture and carry invaders to the lymph nodes or spleen. The name of macrophages comes from Latin meaning "big eaters". Macrophages protect different organs, such as [24]intestines, lungs, [25]liver, and brain. Like dendritic cells, they capture and carry invaders to the lymph organs. These two types of white blood cells are known as [26]scavengers. They eat foreign invaders, **break** them **apart**, and display pieces of the germs known as [27]antigens on their surfaces. The body can then make [28]antibodies to that specific germ, which helps to get rid of that invader faster and remember it in the future. These cells also produce **chemical messengers** that instruct other immune cells to **go into action**.

6   T cells and B cells are also important cells of the immune system. Once antigens are processed and displayed on the surface of macrophages, they can be recognized by T cells which "see" the antigens displayed, [29]coordinate, direct the activity of other types of immune cells, such as macrophages and B cells, and call them into action to fight the [30]intruder. T cells also produce many different chemical messengers in order to communicate effectively with other immune system cells. B cells are another type of immune cell that is turned on by T cells. When a B cell recognizes an antigen, it produces antibodies. An antibody is a protein that **attaches to** an antigen as a key fits a lock. Each antibody matches a specific antigen.

7   When you are exposed to a germ for the first time, it usually takes a while, several weeks to a few months, for your body to produce antibodies to fight it. But if you were exposed to a germ in the past, you will usually still have some B cells (also called memory cells) in your body that recognize or remember the repeat invader. This allows the immune system to go into action right away. This is why people get some diseases, such as ³¹chickenpox or ³²measles, only once. This is also how ³³vaccines work. They introduce your body to an inactive or ³⁴modified form of a particular germ and ³⁵trigger your immune system to produce antibodies to that germ.

Anon. 2021. Understanding the immune system. Thewellproject. Retrieved on July 26, 2022, from Thewellproject website.

(722 words)

Notes

1. (Para. 1) The immune system is made up of cells and organs that protect your body from outside invaders such as bacteria, viruses, fungi, and parasites that can cause infection and disease. 免疫系统由一些细胞和器官组成，保护你的身体免受细菌、病毒、真菌和寄生虫等外部入侵者造成的感染和疾病。
    1）be made up of：由……组成。
    2）句中的 protect... from... 意为"保护……不受……伤害"，from 后可接名词、动名词或代词。

2. (Para. 2) Viruses such as HIV cannot get through normal, healthy and unbroken skin. However, it can get into the body through unbroken mucous membranes. 艾滋病病毒等病毒无法穿透正常、健康、完整的皮肤。然而，它可以通过未破损的黏膜进入人体。
    mucous membranes：黏膜。它是生物体（口腔、胃、肠、尿道等器官）中由上皮组织和结缔组织构成的膜状结构。其结缔组织部分被称为固有层，其上皮组织部分被称为上皮，内有血管和神经，能分泌黏液。黏膜是人体免疫系统的第一道防线。

3. (Para. 4) lymph nodes：淋巴结。淋巴结一般呈肾形或卵圆形，直径一般为 0.1—2.5 厘米。每个淋巴结都由一个纤维状外套膜（capsule）包裹，纤维质延伸至内部形成小梁。其功能类似于过滤器，内部蜂窝状的结构聚集了淋巴球，能够将病毒与细菌摧毁。淋巴结分布在全身，在躯干处相对密集。

4. (Para. 5) Dendritic cells are found mostly in the skin and mucous membranes that protect the openings of the body (e.g. nose, mouth, and throat). 树突状细胞主要存在于保护身体开口（如鼻子、嘴和喉咙）的皮肤和黏膜中。

   1）dendritic cells：树突状细胞，又称树状细胞、树突细胞，是一种存在于哺乳动物的白细胞。它们存在于血液和暴露于环境中的组织中，如皮肤、鼻子、肺、胃和小肠的上皮组织。它们的作用是调节对当前环境刺激的先天和后天免疫反应，其最重要的功能是将抗原处理后呈递给免疫系统的 T 细胞。

   2）句中 openings 为 open 的名词形式，意为"洞口，开口，缺口"。

5. (Para. 5) They eat foreign invaders, break them apart, and display pieces of the germs known as antigens on their surfaces. The body can then make antibodies to that specific germ, which helps to get rid of that invader faster and remember it in the future. 它们吃掉外来入侵者，将其分解，并在自身表面展示被称为抗原的细菌碎片。然后，身体就会产生针对这种特定细菌的抗体，这有助于更快地清除入侵者，并在未来记住它的样子。

6. (Para. 6) Once antigens are processed and displayed on the surface of macrophages, they can be recognized by T cells which "see" the antigens displayed, coordinate, direct the activity of other types of immune cells, such as macrophages and B cells, and call them into action to fight the intruder. 一旦抗原被处理并展示在巨噬细胞表面，它们就会被 T 细胞识别，T 细胞会"看到"展示的抗原，协调、引导巨噬细胞和 B 细胞等其他类型的免疫细胞的活动，并使其运转起来对抗入侵者。

   1）macrophages：巨噬细胞，是由血液中的单核细胞穿出血管后分化而成的。巨噬细胞是形似变形虫的细胞，吞食并处理大型异物、细胞排泄出的老旧废物、衰老的红细胞等，也会前往发生炎症的部位处理异物。它在人体内参与非特异性防卫（先天性免疫）和特异性防卫（细胞免疫），是一种功能很多的白细胞。

   2）T cells：T 细胞，因其来源于胸腺（thymus）而得名。在人体胚胎期和初生期，骨髓中的一部分多能干细胞或前 T 细胞迁移到胸腺内，在胸腺激素的诱导下分化成熟，成为具有免疫活性的 T 细胞。它具有多种生物学功能，如直接杀伤靶细胞，辅助或抑制 B 细胞产生抗体，对特异性抗原和促有丝分裂原的应答反应以及产生细胞因子等。

   3）B cells：B 细胞，因其被发现于鸟类的法布利氏囊（Bursa of Fabricius）而得名。B 细胞的祖细胞存在于胎肝的造血细胞岛（island of hematopoietic cells）中，此后其产生和分化场所逐渐被骨髓所代替。成熟的 B 细胞主要定居于淋巴结皮质浅层的淋巴小结和脾脏的红髓和白髓的淋巴小结内。B 细胞在抗原刺激下可分化为浆细胞，浆细胞可合成和分泌抗体，主要执行机体的体液免疫。

   4）该句中加引号的 see 为比喻说法，意为 T 细胞以某种方式检测、察觉到了抗原。

5）call... into action：使……行动起来；召唤……投入战斗。

7. (Para. 6) An antibody is a protein that attaches to an antigen as a key fits a lock. Each antibody matches a specific antigen. 抗体是一种蛋白质，它附着在抗原上，就像钥匙配锁一样。每个抗体都与特定的抗原相匹配。

该句是比喻说法，正如每把锁都有专门对应的钥匙，每种抗原都有专门匹配的抗体，因为抗原决定簇和抗体分子的超变区之间的空间结构存在互补性。这种特异性是抗原抗体反应的最主要特征，在传染病的诊断与防治方面得到了有效利用。

8. (Para. 7) This allows the immune system to go into action right away. 这（种特性）让免疫系统可以立即投入战斗。

Word List

1. immune [ɪˈmjuːn] *adj.*

that cannot catch or be affected by a particular disease or illness 有免疫力的

2. invader [ɪnˈveɪdər] *n.*

an army or a country, etc. that enters another country, etc. by force in order to take control of it 侵略者；侵入物

3. bacterium [bækˈtɪrɪəm] *n.*

(*pl.* bacteria) a very small organism that exists in large numbers in air, water and soil, and also in living and dead creatures and plants, and is often a cause of disease 细菌

4. fungus [ˈfʌŋɡəs] *n.*

 (*pl.* fungi) a covering of mold or a similar fungus, for example on a plant or wall, that is extremely small and looks like a fine powder 真菌

5. parasite [ˈpærəsaɪt] *n.*

a small animal or plant that lives on or inside another animal or plant and gets its food from it 寄生生物

6. infection [ɪnˈfekʃ(ə)n] *n.*

an illness that is caused by bacteria or a virus and that affects one part of the body 感染

7. pre-cancerous [ˈpriː ˈkænsərəs] *adj.*

displaying characteristics that may develop into cancer 癌症前期的

8. germ [dʒɜːrm] *n.*

a very small living thing that can cause infection and disease 病菌

9. mucous [ˈmjuːkəs] *adj.*

relating to or producing mucus 黏液的；分泌黏液的

10. **membrane** [ˈmembreɪn] *n.*

    a thin layer of skin or tissue that connects or covers parts inside the body 膜

11. **marrow** [ˈmærəʊ] *n.*

    a soft substance that fills the hollow parts of bones 骨髓

12. **lymph** [lɪmf] *n.*

    a clear liquid containing white blood cells that helps to clean the tissues of the body and helps to prevent infections from spreading 淋巴

13. **await** [əˈweɪt] *v.*

    to wait for sb./sth. 等候

14. **node** [nəʊd] *n.*

    a small hard mass of tissue, especially near a joint in the human body 硬结

15. **thymus** [ˈθaɪməs] *n.*

    an organ in the neck that produces lymphocytes (cells to fight infection) 胸腺

16. **spleen** [spliːn] *n.*

    a small organ near the stomach that controls the quality of the blood cells 脾

17. **appendix** [əˈpendɪks] *n.*

    a small closed tube inside your body that is attached to your digestive system 阑尾

18. **armpit** [ˈɑːrmpɪt] *n.*

    the part of the body under the arm where it joins the shoulder 腋窝

19. **abdomen** [ˈæbdəmən] *n.*

    the part of the body below the chest that contains the stomach, intestines, etc. 腹部

20. **groin** [grɔɪn] *n.*

    the part of the body where the legs join at the top including the area around the genitals (sex organs) 腹股沟

21. **filter** [ˈfɪltər] *v.*

    to pass liquid, light, etc. through a special device, especially to remove sth. that is not wanted 过滤

22. **dendritic** [ˌdenˈdrɪtɪk] *adj.*

    of or relating to or resembling a tree 树状的

23. **macrophage** [ˈmækrəfeɪdʒ] *n.*

    a large cell that is able to remove harmful substances from the body, and is found in blood and tissue 巨噬细胞

24. **intestine** [ɪnˈtestɪn] *n.*

    a long tube in your body through which food passes when it has left your stomach 肠

25. **liver** [ˈlɪvər] *n.*

    a large organ in your body which processes your blood and helps to clean unwanted substances out of it 肝脏

26. **scavenger** [ˈskævɪndʒər] *n.*

    anything that removes impurities, refuse, etc. 清道夫

27. **antigen** [ˈæntɪdʒən] *n.*

    a substance that enters the body and helps the production of antibodies 抗原

28. **antibody** [ˈæntɪbɑːdɪ] *n.*

    a substance that the body produces in the blood to fight disease, or as a reaction when certain substances are put into the body 抗体

29. **coordinate** [kəʊˈɔːrdɪneɪt] *v.*

    to organize the different parts of an activity and the people involved in it so that it works well 协调

30. **intruder** [ɪnˈtruːdər] *n.*

    a person who goes into a place where they are not supposed to be 入侵者

31. **chickenpox** [ˈtʃɪkɪnpɑːks] *n.*

    a disease, especially of children, that causes a slight fever and many spots on the skin 水痘

32. **measles** [ˈmiːz(ə)lz] *n.*

    an infectious disease, especially of children, that causes fever and small red spots that cover the whole body 麻疹

33. **vaccine** [vækˈsiːn] *n.*

    a substance that is put into the blood and that protects the body from a disease 疫苗

34. **modify** [ˈmɑːdɪfaɪ] *v.*

    to change sth. slightly, especially in order to make it more suitable for a particular purpose 调整；修改

35. **trigger** [ˈtrɪgər] *v.*

    to make sth. happen suddenly 引起，触发

Chunk List

Collocations

1. **fight off** 抵抗

   These drugs are quite toxic and hinder the body's ability to fight off infection.

   这些药毒性很大，会妨碍身体抗感染的能力。

2. **as follows** 如下

   The winners are as follows: Mary, James, and George.

   获胜者如下：玛丽、詹姆斯、乔治。

3. **take care of** 负责；处理

   David takes care of the marketing side of things.

   大卫负责产品营销方面的事宜。

4. **home base** 基地；总部

   The company's home base is in New York.

   该公司的总部设在纽约。

5. **worn out** 破旧不堪的，报废的

   These shoes are worn out.

   这些鞋破得不能再穿了。

6. **break... apart** 把……分开

   I would break the sentences of a given passage apart.

   我会把一篇文章的句子拆开。

7. **go into action** 采取行动

   They went into action immediately.

   他们立即采取了行动。

8. **attach to** 与……有关联

   No one is suggesting that any health risks attach to this product.

   没有人指出这个产品可能会危害健康。

Idiom and Proverb

9. **get rid of** 摆脱，丢弃

   The problem is getting rid of nuclear waste.

   问题是（如何）处理核废料。

(Sub)Technical Chunks

10. **immune system** 免疫系统

    His immune system completely broke down and he became very ill.

    他的免疫系统彻底崩溃了，他已病入膏肓。

11. **HIV (human immunodeficiency virus)** 人体免疫缺损病毒，艾滋病病毒

    There is no vaccine against HIV infection.

    （现在）还没有防艾滋病病毒传染的疫苗。

12. **white blood cell** 白血球

    The white blood cells attack cells infected with an invader.

    白血球攻击那些受侵并感染的细胞。

13. **bone marrow** 骨髓

    There are 2,000 children worldwide who need a bone marrow transplant.

    全世界有 2 000 名需要骨髓移植的儿童。

14. **lymph node** 淋巴结

    These cells replace normal cells in the marrow and lymph nodes.

    这些细胞取代了骨髓和淋巴结中的正常细胞。

15. **chemical messenger** 化学信使，化学信息素

    Hormones are our bodies' chemical messengers.

    荷尔蒙是我们身体的化学信使。

Text B

How to Boost Your Immune System

1   Your immune system does a remarkable job of defending you against disease-causing [1]microorganisms. But sometimes it fails: A germ invades successfully and makes you sick. Therefore, the idea of boosting your [2]immunity is [3]enticing, but the ability to do so has proved [4]elusive for several reasons. The immune system is precisely a system, not a single [5]entity. To function well, it requires balance and harmony. There is still much that researchers don't know about the [6]intricacies and interconnectedness of the **immune response**. **For now**, there are no scientifically proven direct links between lifestyle and enhanced immune function. But that doesn't mean the effects of certain factors shouldn't be studied. In fact, researchers are exploring

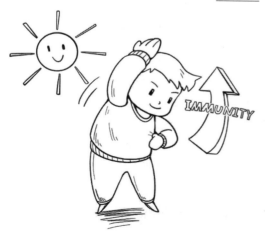

the effects of lifestyle, age, nutrition and other factors on the immune response, both in animals and in humans.

2   Your first line of defense is to choose a healthy lifestyle. Following general good-health guidelines is the single best step you can take toward naturally keeping your immune system working properly. Every part of your body, including your immune system, functions better when protected from environmental [7]assaults and [8]bolstered by healthy-living strategies such as no smoking, eating **a balanced diet**, exercising regularly, maintaining a healthy weight, drinking alcohol only **in** [9]**moderation**, getting adequate sleep, **taking steps** to avoid infection such as washing your hands frequently, cooking meats thoroughly, trying to [10]minimize stress and **keeping pace with** all recommended vaccines.

3   As we age, our immune response capability becomes reduced, which in turn **contributes to** more infections and more cancers. While some people age healthily, the conclusion of many studies is that, compared with younger people, the elderly are more likely to [11]contract **infectious diseases** and, even more importantly, more likely to die from them. [12]**Respiratory infections**, including [13]influenza, the COVID-19 virus and particularly [14]pneumonia are a **leading cause** of death in people over 65 worldwide. No one knows **for sure** why this happens, but some scientists observe that this increased risk [15]correlates with a decrease in T cells, possibly from the thymus [16]atrophying with age and producing fewer T cells to fight off infection. Whether this decrease in thymus function explains the drop in T cells or whether other changes **play a role** is not fully understood. Others are interested in whether the bone marrow becomes less efficient at producing the **stem cells** that **give rise to** the cells of the immune system.

4   A reduction in immune response to infections has been demonstrated by older people's response to vaccines. For example, studies of influenza vaccines have shown that for people over age 65, the vaccine is less effective compared to healthy children over age two. But despite the reduction in [17]efficacy, [18]vaccinations for influenza have significantly lowered the rates of sickness and death in older people when compared with no vaccination.

5   There appears to be a connection between nutrition and immunity in the elderly. A form of [19]malnutrition that is surprisingly common even in [20]affluent countries is known as "[21]micronutrient malnutrition". Micronutrient malnutrition, in which a person is [22]deficient in some essential vitamins and minerals that are obtained from or [23]supplemented by diet, can happen in the elderly. Older people tend to eat less and often have less variety in their diets. One important question is whether **dietary supplements** may help older people maintain a healthier immune system. Older people should discuss this question with their doctor.

6   Like any **fighting force**, the immune system army **marches on its stomach**. Healthy immune system [24]warriors need good and regular [25]nourishment. Scientists have long recognized that people who live in poverty and are [26]malnourished are more [27]vulnerable to infectious diseases. For example, researchers don't know whether any particular dietary factors, such as **processed foods** or high **simple sugar** intake, will [28]adversely affect immune function. There are still relatively few studies of the effects of nutrition on the immune system of humans.

7   There is some evidence that various micronutrient [29]deficiencies, for example, deficiencies of [30]zinc, [31]selenium, iron, [32]copper, **folic acid**, and vitamins A, B6, C, and E, alter immune responses in animals, as measured in the **test tube**. However, the impact of these immune system changes on the health of animals is less clear, and the effect of similar deficiencies on the human immune response has yet to be [33]assessed.

8   So, what can you do? If you don't like vegetables and suspect your diet is not providing you with all your micronutrient needs, taking a daily multivitamin and mineral supplement may bring other health benefits, beyond any possibly beneficial effects on the immune system. But stay alert that taking a [34]mega [35]dose of a single vitamin does not. More is not necessarily better.

Anon. 2021. How to boost your immune system. Health.harvard. Retrieved and adapted on July 11, 2022, from Health.harvard website.

(777 words)

Notes

1. (Para. 1) There is still much that researchers don't know about the intricacies and interconnectedness of the immune response. 对于免疫反应的复杂性和相互关联性，研究人员仍有很多不了解的地方。
    1）句中的 still much that 与常见的 so much that 形式类似，意为"仍有许多……的事物"，that 引导的从句解释 much 代表的具体内容。
    2）interconnectedness 意为"互联性，关联性"，其词根为动词 interconnect（意为"相互连结"）。

2. (Para. 2) Every part of your body, including your immune system, functions

better when protected from environmental assaults and bolstered by healthy-living strategies such as no smoking, eating a balanced diet, exercising regularly, maintaining a healthy weight, drinking alcohol only in moderation, getting adequate sleep, taking steps to avoid infection such as washing your hands frequently, cooking meats thoroughly, trying to minimize stress and keeping pace with all recommended vaccines. 你身体的每个部分，包括你的免疫系统，在健康生活策略的指导下可以免受环境攻击，从而表现更佳，这些策略包括不吸烟、均衡饮食、定期锻炼、保持健康体重、适量饮酒、充足睡眠、采取勤洗手和彻底烹饪肉类等措施避免感染、尝试减小精神压力和接种所有建议接种的疫苗。

3. (Para. 3) While some people age healthily, the conclusion of many studies is that, compared with younger people, the elderly are more likely to contract infectious diseases and, even more importantly, more likely to die from them. 虽然有些人会健康地老去，但许多研究得出结论，与年轻人相比，老年人更可能得传染病，更重要的是，更容易死于传染病。

1）句中的 age 为动词，意为"变老"。

2）句中的 the elderly 为老年人的总称，指代老年人群体。

4. (Para. 3) Whether this decrease in thymus function explains the drop in T cells or whether other changes play a role is not fully understood. 是胸腺功能的下降引发 T 细胞的减少，或是其他变化起了作用，目前还不完全清楚。

1）句中的 whether this decrease... in T cells 和 whether other changes play a role 是并列关系，以 or 连接，意为导致呼吸道感染率增加的原因可能是前者，也可能是后者。

2）play a role：扮演某种角色；发挥某种作用。

5. (Para. 5) A form of malnutrition that is surprisingly common even in affluent countries is known as "micronutrient malnutrition". 有一种甚至在富裕国家也极为普遍的营养不良现象，被称作"微量营养素营养不良"。

micronutrient：微量营养素，指一类生物体需求相对较少，但对生物机体维持正常生理学功能有重要作用的营养物质。对人来说，它主要包含维生素和微量矿物质两大类，其中组成微量矿物质且含量在生物体中低于 0.01% 的元素又被称为"微量元素"。

6. (Para. 6) For example, researchers don't know whether any particular dietary factors, such as processed foods or high simple sugar intake, will adversely affect immune function. 例如，研究人员不知道特定的饮食因素，如加工食品或高单糖摄入量，是否会对免疫功能产生不利影响。

simple sugar：单糖，是最简形式的糖，为糖类的最基本单元，包括葡萄糖、半乳糖和果糖等。作为食物的淀粉（多糖）和蔗糖（双糖）都需要人或动物体内的酶将其分解成单糖才能吸收，食品工业中添加的游离糖多为单糖和双糖，过量食用可能造成营养不良、体重增长等问题。

7. (Para. 7) There is some evidence that various micronutrient deficiencies, for example, deficiencies of zinc, selenium, iron, copper, folic acid, and vitamins A, B6, C, and E, alter immune responses in animals, as measured in the test tube. 通过试管实验测算，有证据表明，锌、硒、铁、铜、叶酸、维生素 A、维生素 B6、维生素 C、维生素 E 等多种微量营养素的缺乏会改变动物机体的免疫反应。

8. (Para. 8) But stay alert that taking a mega dose of a single vitamin does not. More is not necessarily better. 但是注意，摄入大量的同一种维生素并不能（对免疫系统更有益）。（摄入）更多不一定效果更好。

1）"But stay alert…" 一句的从句部分内容有省略，完整意思为 taking a… vitamin does not bring other health benefits。

2）"More is not necessarily better." 一句的字面意思为 "更多不一定更好。" 需结合语境来理解这句话，本句中的 more 指代 more single vitamin，better 指代 better effects on the immune system。

Word List

1. **microorganism** [ˌmaɪkrəʊˈɔːrgənɪzəm] *n.*
   a very small living thing which you can only see if you use a microscope 微生物

2. **immunity** [ɪˈmjuːnətɪ] *n.*
   the body's ability to avoid or not be affected by infection and disease 免疫力

3. **enticing** [ɪnˈtaɪsɪŋ] *adj.*
   (of sth.) so attractive and interesting that you want to have or know more about it 诱人的

4. **elusive** [ɪˈluːsɪv] *adj.*
   difficult to find, define, or achieve 难找的；难以解释的；难以达到的

5. **entity** [ˈentətɪ] *n.*
   sth. that exists separately from other things and has its own identity 实体

6. **intricacy** [ˈɪntrɪkəsɪ] *n.*
   the complicated parts or details of sth. 错综复杂的事物或细节

7. **assault** [əˈsɔːlt] *n.*
   the act of attacking a building, an area, etc. in order to take control of it 袭击

8. **bolster** [ˈbəʊlstər] *v.*
   to improve sth. or make it stronger 改善；加强

9. **moderation** [ˌmɑːdəˈreɪʃ(ə)n] *n.*

    the quality of being reasonable and not being extreme 适度

10. **minimize** [ˈmɪnɪmaɪz] *v.*

    to reduce sth., especially sth. bad, to the lowest possible level 使某物减少到最低限度

11. **contract** [kənˈtrækt] *v.*

    to get an illness 感染

12. **respiratory** [ˈrespərətɔːrɪ] *adj.*

    connected with breathing 呼吸的

13. **influenza** [ˌɪnfluˈenzə] *n.*

    an infectious disease like a very bad cold, that causes fever, pains and weakness 流行性感冒

14. **pneumonia** [nuːˈməʊnɪə] *n.*

    a serious illness affecting one or both lungs that makes breathing difficult 肺炎

15. **correlate** [ˈkɔːrəˌleɪt] *v.*

    to have a mutual relationship or connection, in which one thing affects or depends on another 相关

16. **atrophy** [ˈætrəfɪ] *v.*

    to decrease in size or strength, often as a result of an illness 萎缩

17. **efficacy** [ˈefɪkəsɪ] *n.*

    the ability of sth., especially a drug or a medical treatment, to produce the results that are wanted 功效

18. **vaccination** [ˌvæksɪˈneɪʃ(ə)n] *n.*

    the act or practice of giving a person or an animal a substance, especially by injecting it, in order to protect them against a disease 接种疫苗

19. **malnutrition** [ˌmælnuˈtrɪʃ(ə)n] *n.*

    a poor condition of health caused by a lack of food or a lack of the right type of food 营养不良

20. **affluent** [ˈæfluənt] *adj.*

    having a lot of money and a good standard of living 富裕的

21. **micronutrient** [ˌmaɪkrəʊˈnjuːtrɪənt] *n.*

    any substance, such as a vitamin, essential for healthy growth and development but required only in minute amounts 微量营养元素

22. **deficient** [dɪˈfɪʃ(ə)nt] *adj.*

    not having enough of sth., especially sth. that is essential 缺乏的，不足的

23. **supplement** [ˈsʌplɪment] *v.*

    to add sth. to sth. in order to improve it or make it more complete 补充

24. **warrior** [ˈwɔːrɪər] *n.*

    a person who fights in a battle or war 武士，勇士

25. **nourishment** [ˈnɜːrɪʃmənt] *n.*

    food that is needed to stay alive, grow and stay healthy 营养

26. **malnourished** [ˌmælˈnɜːrɪʃt] *adj.*

    in bad health because of a lack of food or a lack of the right type of food 营养不良的

27. **vulnerable** [ˈvʌlnərəb(ə)l] *adj.*

    more likely to get a disease than other people, animals, or plants 容易患病的

28. **adversely** [ədˈvɜːrslɪ] *adv.*

    in a way that is bad or harmful 不利地，有害地

29. **deficiency** [dɪˈfɪʃ(ə)nsɪ] *n.*

    the state of not having, or not having enough of sth. that is essential 缺乏，不足

30. **zinc** [zɪŋk] *n.*

    a trace element in the diet; a component of several enzymes 锌

31. **selenium** [səˈliːnɪəm] *n.*

    a chemical element; an essential mineral nutrient in the seafood, kidney, and liver 硒

32. **copper** [ˈkɑːpər] *n.*

    a chemical element necessary for bone and blood formation 铜

33. **assess** [əˈses] *v.*

    to make a judgmentt about the nature or quality of sb./sth. 评估

34. **mega** [ˈmegə] *adj.*

    very large or impressive 巨大的；极佳的

35. **dose** [dəʊs] *n.*

    an amount of a medicine or a drug that is taken once, or regularly over a period of time 剂量；一剂

Chunk List

Collocations

1. **for now** 目前；暂时

Although the shooting has stopped for now, the destruction left behind is enormous.

虽然枪战目前已停止，但造成的破坏是极大的。

2. **in moderation** 适中；有节制

Alcohol should only be taken in moderation.

酒只可适量饮用。

3. **take steps** 采取措施

We are taking steps to prevent pollution.

我们正在采取措施防止污染。

4. **contribute to** 是……的一个原因

The research showed that smoking contributes to heart disease.

这项研究表明，吸烟会导致心脏疾病。

5. **leading cause** 主要原因

Lack of physical exercise is the leading cause of obesity in young students.

缺乏体育锻炼是青少年学生肥胖的主要原因。

6. **for sure** 确定；毫无疑问地

No one knows for sure what happened.

谁也不确定究竟发生了什么事。

7. **play a role** 发挥作用

The media plays a major role in influencing people's opinions.

媒体在影响舆论方面发挥着重要作用。

8. **fighting force** 战斗部队

Four thousand troops have been reorganized into a fighting force.

4 000 名士兵被重组成为一支战斗部队。

Idioms and Proverbs

9. **keep pace with** 与……保持同步

Until now, wage increases have always kept pace with inflation.

到目前为止，工资的增长与通货膨胀始终保持同步。

10. **give rise to** 引起，导致

Tourism, however, gives rise to a number of problems.

然而，旅游业引起了许多问题。

11. **march on its stomach** 行军靠肚皮（给养充足才能战斗）

An army marches on its stomach.

给养充足的士兵才能（很好地）战斗。

(Sub)Technical Chunks

12. **immune response** 免疫反应

    It is hoped that the procedure will trigger an immune response that will wipe out HIV-infected cells.

    希望这一治疗会激发免疫反应，清除感染了艾滋病病毒的细胞。

13. **a balanced diet** 均衡饮食

    He cut down on coffee and cigarettes, and ate a balanced diet.

    他少喝咖啡，少抽烟，饮食均衡。

14. **infectious disease** 传染病

    Those suffering from infectious diseases were separated from the other patients.

    传染病患者同其他病人隔离开来。

15. **respiratory infection** 呼吸道感染

    Repeated respiratory infection is a common disease in children.

    反复呼吸道感染是儿童的常见病。

16. **stem cell** 干细胞

    Stem cell research is supported by many doctors.

    干细胞研究得到很多医生的支持。

17. **dietary supplement** 膳食补充剂

    Such disorders are generally treated with dietary supplements and drugs.

    这类疾病通常是用膳食补充剂和药物来治疗。

18. **processed food** 加工食品

    I recommend that you avoid processed foods whenever possible.

    我建议你尽量不要食用加工食品。

19. **simple sugar** 单糖

    Glucose is a simple sugar which gives you energy.

    葡萄糖是一种提供能量的单糖。

20. **folic acid** 叶酸

    Iron and folic acid supplements are frequently given to pregnant women.

    孕妇经常服用铁和叶酸补充剂。

21. **test tube** 试管

    Take care not to break the test tube!

    当心别把试管打碎了！

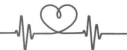

Part 3 Post-reading Exercises

3.1 Read and Answer

3.1.1 *Directions: Read Text A in Part 2 and choose the best answers to the following questions.*

1. What can cause infection and disease in a person's body?
   A. Fungi.
   B. Bacteria.
   C. Parasites.
   D. All of the above.

2. Which of the following is true about the immune system?
   A. It is only made up of cells.
   B. It can't get rid of cancerous cells.
   C. It can't protect you from viruses.
   D. It can keep you healthy.

3. Which of the following facts about skin is NOT mentioned?
   A. It keeps bacteria and viruses from entering the body.
   B. It is the single and best line of defense against germs.
   C. It is the single largest organ of the body.
   D. Normal, healthy and unbroken skin can stop HIV viruses.

4. How does the immune system help if germs get inside the body?
   A. The red blood cells will defend the body from invaders.
   B. The internal parts of the immune system such as the white blood cells will work.
   C. The bone marrow will help get rid of dangerous abnormal cells.
   D. Cells in the neck will work to defend against invaders.

5. Lymph nodes are located in the following body parts EXCEPT the _____.
   A. wrist   B. neck
   C. armpit   D. abdomen

6. What do you know about spleen according to the text?
   A. It is about the size of two adult fists.
   B. It is located in the upper right of the belly.
   C. It plays a key role in getting rid of unuseful white blood cells.
   D. It has nothing to do with the immune system.

7. Which of the following are NOT important cells of the immune system?
   A. Dendritic cells.
   B. T cells.
   C. Liver cells.
   D. B cells.

8. Why are dendritic cells and macrophages called "scavengers" in Paragraph 5?
   A. Because they eat foreign invaders and break them apart.
   B. Because they protect the openings of the body.
   C. Because they carry invaders to the lymph organs.
   D. Because they produce chemical messengers.

9. From the text, we can infer that _____.
   A. the immune system only includes four kinds of cells
   B. your body can produce antibodies instantly when you are exposed to a germ
   C. you may get chickenpox twice
   D. some cells of the immune system work together to protect your body

10. What is the main idea of this text?
   A. How viruses get inside your body.
   B. An introduction to the immune system.
   C. The importance of skin cells.
   D. How T cells and B cells work to fight against viruses.

3.1.2 Directions: *Read Text B in Part 2 and finish the following exercises. Write T for True, F for False, or NG for Not Given in the brackets before the statements based on the instructions below.*

True	*if the statement agrees with the claims of the author;*
False	*if the statement contradicts the claims of the author;*
Not Given	*if it is impossible to say what the author thinks about it.*

(   ) 1. Your immune system may fail sometimes.

(   ) 2. It has been proven that lifestyles can directly enhance immune functions.

(   ) 3. A healthy lifestyle does help keep your immune system work properly.

(   ) 4. The immune system becomes weaker as age increases.

(   ) 5. The decrease in T cells has something to do with some diseases that cause death in older people.

(   ) 6. Vaccinations for influenza have no positive effect on older people.

(   ) 7. Older people may often have micronutrient malnutrition due to less variety in their diets.

( ) 8. It is found that people living in poverty with insufficient nutrition are more likely to contract infectious diseases.

( ) 9. There will be some experiments about the effect of micronutrient deficiencies on the health of animals.

( ) 10. Proper supplementation of multivitamins might have good health benefits.

3.2 Guess and Choose

Directions: Figure out the meanings of the following medical affixes and choose the best answer from the four choices marked A, B, C and D.

1. immune, immuno ( )
   A. disease-free   B. imitate   C. beyond   D. immerse

2. cyt, cyte, cyto ( )
   A. cynic   B. cynical   C. cynicism   D. cell

3. lymph, lympho ( )
   A. a solid tissue in white blood cells
   B. a clear liquid containing white blood cells
   C. air sacs containing red blood cells
   D. a soft tissue containing red blood cells

4. lip, lipo ( )
   A. lip of mouth   B. lippy   C. fat   D. lipped

5. thyr, thyro ( )
   A. thyme   B. thymus   C. thyroid   D. thyself

6. coron, corona, coronary ( )
   A. crown   B. colon   C. coral   D. core

7. bronch, bronchi, broncho ( )
   A. branch   B. bronchus   C. brown   D. brochure

8. derm, derma, dermat, dermato, dermo ( )
   A. demo   B. democrat   C. skin   D. democracy

9. anti ( )
   A. antenna   B. antique   C. anthem   D. against

10. ase ( )
    A. enzyme   B. assess   C. assemble   D. asset

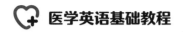
3.3 Read and Think

Directions: Read the following medical words built with the medical affixes from Exercise 3.2 and write down their Chinese equivalents in the table below.

Terminology	Chinese Equivalents	Terminology	Chinese Equivalents
immune		immunity	
cytoblast		cytology	
lymphocyte		lymphoid	
lipase		lipoprotein	
thyroid		thyroxine	
corona		coronary	
bronchitis		bronchus	
dermatology		dermatitis	
antibody		antigen	
protease		diastase	

3.4 Match and Fill

3.4.1 *Directions: Match the medical terms (a–j) in the box below with their definitions (1–10).*

a. immune	b. parasite	c. germ	d. contract	e. antibody
f. chickenpox	g. vaccine	h. dose	i. respiratory	j. malnutrition

(   ) **1.** any organism capable of causing disease

(   ) **2.** a substance that the body produces in the blood to fight diseases, or as a reaction when certain substances are put into the body

(   ) **3.** an amount of a medicine or a drug that is taken once, or regularly over a period of time

(   ) **4.** free from the possibility of acquiring a given infectious disease

(   ) **5.** relating to breathing

(   ) **6.** a disease, especially of children, that causes a slight fever and many spots on the skin

(   ) **7.** an organism that lives on or in another and draws its nourishment therefrom

(   ) **8.** lack of proper nutrition; inadequate or unbalanced nutrition

(　　) 9. a substance that is put into the blood and that protects the body from a disease

(　　) 10. to get an illness by infection

3.4.2 Directions: *Make good use of the medical terms you learned from Exercise 3.4.1 and fill in the blanks in the sentences below. Change the form where necessary.*

1. It is likely to _____ COVID-19 if you don't wear face masks in crowded places.

2. Pregnancy suppresses the maternal _____ system, increasing susceptibility to infections by common microbes.

3. These gases would seriously damage the patient's _____ system.

4. People with low levels of a particular type of _____ tend to have more heart attacks.

5. Hunger and _____ are a cause, not just a result, of poverty.

6. A(n) _____ is an organism that feeds on other organisms.

7. The search for a new _____ will take priority over all other medical research.

8. In most cases, getting _____ once means you will not get it again.

9. It is dangerous to exceed the recommended _____.

10. Dirty hands can be a breeding ground for _____.

3.5 Fill and Translate

3.5.1 Directions: *Choose the correct medical words from the box below to fill in the gaps (1–10) of the passage concerning the immune system. Change the form where necessary.*

marrow	cell	defend	swell	primary
filter	expose	allergic	organ	antibody

The immune system is constantly working hard to (1) _____ you, but you can lend a helping hand by caring for your immune health from the inside out. The best place to start is by learning more about how the immune system actually works. The immune system's (2) _____ job is to serve as the body's protection system. Its overall function is to both prevent and limit infections by recognizing danger cues and distinguishing between normal, healthy, and unhealthy cells. Once a danger signal is recognized, the immune system responds to address the problem.

Problems like an infection or illness can occur when a sufficient immune response cannot be activated. (3) _____ reactions or autoimmune diseases, on the other hand, happen when an immune response is activated without a real threat, or isn't turned off once danger passes. The immune system is a vast and incredible system of the smallest cells and largest organs, all working together to protect you. Some of the main immune system (4) _____ are the skin, which includes mucous membranes; the lymphatic system, which includes the bone (5) _____, tonsils (扁桃体), lymph nodes, and spleen; and your stomach and gut.

Let's talk a bit about a few immune system standouts. The lymph nodes, which are found all over your body, may (6) _____ up when you're feeling sick. They work as a(n) (7) _____ system to kill germs and bacteria. The bone marrow is the "manufacturing center" for red and white blood (8) _____; it makes millions of them per day. Your mucous membranes help defend you in a variety of ways; mucus and tiny hairs in your nose trap bacteria and help you sneeze, for example. Even your sweat can play defense against germs! Stomach acid kills bacteria, and a great deal of immune tissue is found in the gut itself. These organs and cells make up the two immune systems: the innate immune system and the acquired immune system. The innate immune system is the first to respond when it recognizes danger. The cells of the innate immune system engulf the invader and work to kill it. The innate system then sends information from the frontlines to the acquired immune system to produce targeted cells, called (9) _____, to protect against a specific invader. This means that after initial (10) _____ to a given invader or sickness, the body remembers it and can respond accordingly in the future. When your immune system is working properly, your body can easily fend off sicknesses and bounce back from colds.

3.5.2 Directions: Translate the underlined sentences from the passage above.

1. Its overall function is to both prevent and limit infections by recognizing danger cues and distinguishing between normal, healthy, and unhealthy cells.

   _____

   _____

2. Problems like an infection or illness can occur when a sufficient immune response cannot be activated.

   _____

   _____

3. The immune system is a vast and incredible system of the smallest cells and largest organs, all working together to protect you.

_____

_____

4. These organs and cells make up the two immune systems: the innate immune system and the acquired immune system.

_____

_____

5. When your immune system is working properly, your body can easily fend off sicknesses and bounce back from colds.

_____

_____

3.6 Speak and Write

3.6.1 Directions: Discuss with your group members the phenomenon described in Topic 1 below, and select a representative to report your main ideas to the class.

Topic 1

If a child has frequent infections, the worst thing to do is administer him lots of antibiotics. The excessive use of these medications may lead to antibiotic resistance, and major consequences may occur just when they might be helpful to cure serious diseases. The antibiotic resistance is the perfect example to understand how the immune system may be damaged, yet there are also specific factors that may damage the immune system. What may damage or weaken the immune system? Discuss with your partners about it and analyze the reasons.

3.6.2 Directions: Discuss with your group members the phenomenon described in Topic 2 below, and write an essay in about 160 words, entitled "The Effects of a Healthy Lifestyle on the Immune System".

Topic 2

Winter is a "cold and flu season". Almost every mother has said it: "Wear a jacket or you'll catch a cold!" Even though you may have taken your flu shot and have been vaccinated, chances are, you do get these diseases. The immune system is your body's natural defense against microorganisms that cause diseases. There are times, however, when the system fails and germs are able to invade your body, ultimately making you sick. To avoid this, it is important to maintain good health. The simplest way to strengthen your immune system is to adopt a healthy lifestyle. Do you have any tips on that, especially when the winter season comes? Give evidence to support your view.

Part 4 Mini-lecture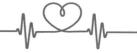

A Small Experiment

Let's begin this series of mini-lectures with a small translation exercise. Please put the following three sentences from Chinese into English.

1. 她存不住钱。

2. 他面试没有成功，还认为室友的安慰是假惺惺的。

3. 杰克对经理感到很失望，觉得自己的创意对经理来讲就是对牛弹琴。

4. 我立刻在网上下了订单，因为这套家具的口碑很好而且物有所值。

Now that you've done the job, we will provide you with, for each Chinese sentence, two English equivalents, the first of which is typical of the work from Chinese learners of English, and the second has been offered by native English speakers.

1. 她存不住钱。

- She can't save money.
- *Money burns a hole in her pocket.*

2. 他面试没有成功，还认为室友的安慰是假惺惺的。
   - He failed on the job interview and thought his roommate's comfort is fake.
   - *He failed on the job interview and thought his roommate's comfort is crocodile tears.*

3. 杰克对经理感到很失望，觉得自己的创意对经理来讲就是对牛弹琴。
   - Jack feels very disappointed and thinks his creativity is like playing the piano before a cow.
   - *Jack is disappointed at the manager and believes that his creativity is like casting pearls before swine.*

4. 我立刻在网上下了订单，因为这套家具的口碑很好而且物有所值。
   - I immediately made an order on the Internet, because the set of furniture has a good reputation and the value of the furniture is equal to the price.
   - *I immediately placed an order online, because I learned this set of furniture by word of mouth and knew it gives good value for money.*

After the above comparison and contrast, it's likely that we have reached a consensus that the second version of the translation is more vivid and idiomatic. However, if you carefully examine the words used, you will find there're no new single words at all. To put it another way, the reason why the native English translators win an upper hand is not that they have used more difficult or challenging words. The recipe for their success is the use of chunks. By "chunks", we mean a cluster or string of words which are different from the long lists of single words you have learned for so many years. Idioms such as "burn a hole in the pocket" instantly conjure up a picture in one's mind that the pocket loses the function of holding things. So is "crocodile tears". "Cast pearls before swine" is another English chunk which means even if you give somebody something very valuable, he/she can not appreciate its value, while "play the piano before a cow" is not only a word-for-word translation, but may also lead to a question of "Why not an ox?"; "place an order" "word of mouth" "give good value for money" are all normal and correct collocations, while "make an order" is Chinglish (Chinese English). It's worth mentioning that the average native speaker knows hundreds of thousands of chunks which may be used in ongoing conversations to achieve the degree of real-time fluency that is taken for granted, and that would not be attainable otherwise.

As an advanced learner of English (you are "advanced" simply because you may have already spent more than a decade learning English), you are suggested to pay more attention to the acquisition of chunks, instead of those single and individual words. It has been proven to be an efficient and effective means of improving your productive competence such as speaking, writing, interpreting and translating. Therefore, at the very beginning of the mini-lecture series in this coursebook, we endeavor to get this message across, loud and clear, to all of you. The importance of learning chunks and the methods of effectively learning chunks will be discussed in detail in the following mini-lectures which comprise the last part of each chapter in this coursebook. Stay tuned.

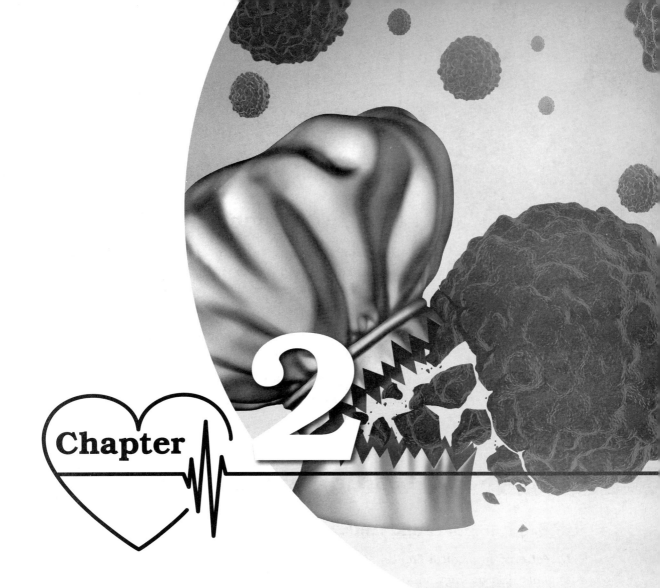

Chapter **2**

Preventive Medicine

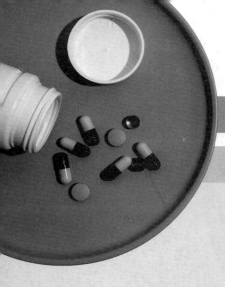

Chapter 2

Preventive Medicine

Learning Objectives

- to master some basic skills to build medical words with affixes concerning preventive medicine and to expand accurate usage of amphibious words in both general and medical contexts;

- to improve comprehensive linguistic abilities to discuss preventive medicine;

- to increase awareness of the importance of fostering a good attitude to and habits of preventing an illness.

Part 1   Pre-reading Tasks

Task 1   Compare and Contrast

*Directions: In medical English, **amphibious words**, a term derived from amphibious animals such as frogs and toads that can live both on land and in water, have flexible meanings in both general contexts and medical contexts. Please consult your dictionaries, write down the Chinese equivalents of the amphibious words in the table below, and pay attention to their different meanings used as **general expressions (GE)** and **medical expressions (ME)** respectively. The first one is exemplified for you to follow.*

Amphibious Words	GE	ME
acquired	习得的	后天的，获得性的
activity		
colon		
congestion		
focus		
isolate		

(Continued)

Amphibious Words	GE	ME
obstruction		
operation		
period		
section		

Task 2 Read and Translate

Directions: Please read the following 10 pairs of sentences, and keep an eye on the 10 amphibious words you learned from the table in Task 1, which are interpreted differently as GE and ME. Translate the English sentences into Chinese.

1. Having read the book, she will be able to pass on the <u>acquired</u> knowledge to trainee teachers. (GE)

   _____

   _____

   <u>Acquired</u> and genetic sources of excessive blood clotting are not related but a person can have both. (ME)

   _____

   _____

2. We plan to widen the scope of our existing <u>activities</u> by offering more language courses. (GE)

   _____

   _____

   In the mixed lymphocyte culture, the antibody exhibited desirable immunosuppressive <u>activity</u>. (ME)

   _____

   _____

3. <u>Colons</u> separate hours, minutes, and seconds, although all need not be specified. (GE)

   _____

   _____

The tumor encircles the colon and infiltrates into the wall. (ME)

_____

_____

4. The problems of traffic congestion will not disappear in a hurry at peak time. (GE)

_____

_____

About 95% of patients with acute heart failure show fluid overload and tissue congestion. (ME)

_____

_____

5. Students should resist the temptation and focus on study. (GE)

_____

_____

A benign tumor can be removed by surgery and its focus will disappear after it. (ME)

_____

_____

6. Political influence is being used to shape public opinion and isolate critics. (GE)

_____

_____

Patients will be isolated from other people for between three days and one month after treatment. (ME)

_____

_____

7. The traffic congestion and obstruction is the urgent problem to be considered and addressed. (GE)

_____

_____

Acute colon obstruction caused by large intestinal cancer is a difficult and disputed surgical problem. (ME)

_____

_____

8. All transport operations, whether by sea, rail or road, are closely monitored at all times. (GE)

    _____

    _____

    He had an operation to remove an obstruction in his throat. (ME)

    _____

    _____

9. He will remain head of state during the period of transition to democracy. (GE)

    _____

    _____

    Young girls had better not swim and drink cold coke during their monthly period. (ME)

    _____

    _____

10. The brochure is divided into two sections, dealing firstly with basic courses and secondly with advanced ones. (GE)

    _____

    _____

    The surgery involves making a tiny section in her trachea. (ME)

    _____

    _____

Task 3 Lead-in Questions

Directions: Read the questions below and answer them in details.

1. Have you ever heard about a famous saying "the best doctor cures no diseases"? What's your personal interpretation of this saying?

   _____

   _____

2. Do you know the words "probiotics" and "microbiome"? Consult a dictionary if you don't. Do you eat gut probiotics to prevent intestinal diseases?

   _____

   _____

3. Many people hold the belief that health means the absence of disease. Do you agree? Why or why not?

   _____

   _____

4. Do you often stay up late at night? If so, what do you think of the impact of this habit on your health?

   _____

   _____

Part 2 Texts

Text A

Preventive Health Care and Its Value

1   For too long, the US health care industry has been focused on treating illnesses **after the fact**, which means that patient care is **more** [1]reactive **than** [2]proactive, leading to two major problems. The first is that health care issues are left to grow in [3]severity before they're treated, which is not [4]optimal for the patient. The second is that more severe health care issues generally [5]**equate to** treatment being more expensive for patients and health care providers.

2   These two issues have brought the importance of preventive health care **to the** ⁶forefront of the industry. To understand what preventive health care is and why it matters to patients, it's essential to understand that preventive health care is a proactive approach to ⁷addressing health care concerns. It attempts to deal with

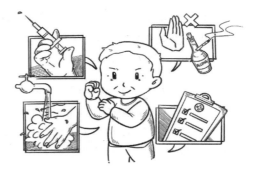

issues before an **emergency room** visit is required or an illness has progressed past the point of effective treatment.

3   As health care ⁸professionals progress through their careers, pursuing advanced education, such as a Healthcare **MBA**, can help them stay **up to date** with industry trends and medical ⁹breakthroughs while **tailoring** their education **to** what will be happening in the future of health care.

4   Anyone interested in getting **a better grasp on** what preventive health care is should explore the many preventive care examples in the health care field today. The concept behind preventive health care is to be proactive rather than reactive, which means patients start **taking advantage of** the resources available to them as early as possible to avoid ¹⁰critical health issues. The following are some of the most common preventive care examples.

5   The most widely known preventive care examples are vaccines, ¹¹screenings and tests administered during ¹²checkups to identify and prevent health issues. The **flu shot** and vaccines that protect against measles, ¹³mumps, ¹⁴polio and COVID-19 are just a few examples of preventive health care measures offered in the US. Health care providers also check ¹⁵cholesterol levels, **blood pressure** and other ¹⁶diagnostics as a proactive measure during checkups.

6   **When it comes to** disease and illness, public health measures are excellent examples of preventive care. Public health is the ¹⁷promotion of wellness through education and the encouragement of healthy behaviors. There are several public health programs—for both children and adults—that stress the importance of diet and exercise; the dangers of smoking, drugs and alcohol; and the necessity of washing our hands.

7   With the number of seniors growing ¹⁸dramatically, the field of **genetic testing** and its ability to ¹⁹map a patient's future health can ²⁰potentially increase **life expectancy** and enhance the quality of life. Doctors are increasingly using genetic testing to [21]diagnose **genetic** [22]**disorders** and predict the risks of developing common diseases. This approach can make a patient aware of potential health issues before it's too late to treat them.

8　To test the success and [23]viability of genetic testing as it relates to preventive health care, the **Centers for Disease Control and Prevention** [24]launched the EGAPP (Evaluation of [25]Genomic Applications in Practice and Prevention) [26]initiative. It aims to "establish and test a systematic, evidence-based process for evaluating genetic tests and other applications of genomic technology that are **in transition from** research **to** [27]clinical and public health practice".

9　Not only is EGAPP **crucial to** advancing the science involved in genetic testing, but the information it collects will be used by health care providers and payers, as well as policymakers. Genetic testing as it relates to preventive health care must involve safe and effective procedures to realize its vast potential to help patients.

10　No one likes going to the doctor. To many, seeing a physician means you have a problem, something is wrong, or you're sick. It's why you [28]self-medicate a [29]nasty cold with a hot bath and honey-lemon tea, or ignore that weird [30]bump on your neck because you had one last year and it **went away on its own**. While the [31]odds may **be on your side**, everyone faces illness **at one point** in his/her life. And though a visit to your **GP** may seem unnecessary or stressful, preventive checkups save millions of lives and billions of dollars each year. According to the American Public Health Association (APHA), "if preventive health screenings were to increase by 90%, then several billion dollars usually spent on health care would be saved each year in the United States alone".

11　Preventive health care saves billions of dollars and millions of lives each year. Professionals with health care degrees and careers [32]facilitate this care through education, screenings, and early [33]intervention for [34]chronic and [35]acute [36]conditions. Nevertheless, not all illnesses are preventable, but taking care of ourselves in specific ways can help reduce our chances of getting sick.

Anon. 2021. What is preventive healthcare? Healthcaremba. Retrieved and adapted on August 11, 2022, from Healthcaremba website.
Sutherland, K. 2020. The value of preventive health: Degrees & careers in early care. Edumed. Retrieved and adapted on August 13, 2022, from Edumed website.

(777 words)

Notes

1. (Para. 1) For too long, the US health care industry has been focused on treating illnesses after the fact, which means that patient care is more reactive than proactive, leading to two major problems. 长期以来，美国医疗保健行业一直专注于治疗已发现的疾病，也就是说对患者的护理更多是被动反应的，而不是主动预防的，这导致了两个主要问题。

2. (Para. 2) To understand what preventive health care is and why it matters to patients, it's essential to understand that preventive health care is a proactive approach to addressing health care concerns. 为了理解什么是预防性保健以及为什么它对患者很重要，我们必须明白，预防性保健是一种应对健康问题时主动预防的方法。

an approach to：（处理某事的）途径，方法。其后接名词或动名词。

3. (Para. 4) The concept behind preventive health care is to be proactive rather than reactive, which means patients start taking advantage of the resources available to them as early as possible to avoid critical health issues. 预防性保健的理念是主动预防，而不是被动反应，患者应尽早开始利用可用的资源，以避免严重的健康问题。

1）take advantage of：利用……的优势。

2）critical issue：关键问题，重要问题。

4. (Para. 5) The most widely known preventive care examples are vaccines, screenings and tests administered during checkups to identify and prevent health issues. 最广为人知的预防性保健的例子有疫苗、筛查和体检期间为确诊和预防健康问题而进行的化验等。

1）vaccine：疫苗。疫苗接种是一种简单、安全和有效的预防疾病的方法，利用身体的天然防御机制来建立对特定感染的抵抗力，并增强免疫系统。疫苗可以训练人的免疫系统像暴露在疾病中一样产生抗体。疫苗只含有灭活或致病力显著下降的减毒活病毒或细菌，因此不会导致疾病或并发症。大多数疫苗通过注射接种，也有些是口服或鼻喷式。

2）screening：筛检，又称筛查，即运用快速简便的实验检查或其他手段，从表面健康的人群中发现那些未被识别的可疑病人或有缺陷者。筛检试验不是诊断试验，仅是一个初步检查，对筛检试验阳性和可疑阳性的人必须进行进一步的确诊检查。筛查可以使临床前期或临床初期的可疑病人得到早诊、早治，及时发现某些疾病的高危个体，或了解疾病的患病率及其趋势，为公共卫生决策提供科学依据等。

5. (Para. 7) This approach can make a patient aware of potential health issues before it's too late to treat them. 这种方法可以让病人发现潜在的健康问题，在为时已晚之前治疗疾病。

make sb. aware of：令某人意识到 / 发现。

6　(Para. 8) It aims to "establish and test a systematic, evidence-based process for evaluating genetic tests and other applications of genomic technology that are in transition from research to clinical and public health practice". 它的目标是"建立和测试一个系统、循证的流程，以评估正在从科研过渡到临床和公共卫生实践的基因检测和其他基因组技术的应用"。

7.　(Para. 9) Genetic testing as it relates to preventive health care must involve safe and effective procedures to realize its vast potential to help patients. 基因检测与预防性保健关系紧密，因此必须采用安全有效的程序，以实现其帮助患者的巨大潜能。

genetic testing：基因检测，是通过血液、其他体液或细胞对 DNA 进行检测，分析它所含有的基因类型和基因缺陷及其表达功能是否正常的一种方法。它可以使人们了解自己的基因信息，也可以用于疾病风险的预测。应用最广泛的基因检测是新生儿遗传性疾病的检测、遗传疾病的诊断和某些常见病的辅助诊断。

8.　(Para. 10) It's why you self-medicate a nasty cold with a hot bath and honey-lemon tea, or ignore that weird bump on your neck because you had one last year and it went away on its own. 这也是为什么你会洗个热水澡、喝杯蜂蜜柠檬茶来自我治疗重感冒，或者直接忽略脖子上奇怪的肿块，因为你去年长过这样的肿块而且它自己消失了。

Word List

1.　**reactive** [rɪ'æktɪv] *adj.*
    acting in response to a situation rather than creating or controlling it 被动反应的，回应性的

2.　**proactive** [ˌprəʊ'æktɪv] *adj.*
    controlling a situation by making things happen rather than waiting for things to happen and then reacting to them 积极主动的；先发制人的

3.　**severity** [sɪ'verətɪ] *n.*
    the quality or state of being severe 严重性

4.　**optimal** ['ɑːptɪm(ə)l] *adj.*
    (also optimum) most desirable or satisfactory 最优的

5.　**equate** [ɪ'kweɪt] *v.*
    (of one thing) to be the same as or equivalent to (another) 等同于

6.　**forefront** ['fɔːrfrʌnt] *n.*
    the leading or most important position or place 最前列；最重要的位置

7. **address** [ə'dres] *v.*

   to think about a problem or a situation and decide how you are going to deal with it 设法解决，处理

8. **professional** [prə'feʃ(ə)n(ə)l] *n.*

   a person who does a job that needs special training and a high level of education 专业人士

9. **breakthrough** ['breɪkθruː] *n.*

   an important development that may lead to an agreement or achievement 突破

10. **critical** ['krɪtɪk(ə)l] *adj.*

    serious and possibly dangerous 严重的；可能有危险的

11. **screening** ['skriːnɪŋ] *n.*

    the testing or examining of a large number of people or things for disease, faults, etc. 筛查

12. **checkup** ['tʃeɪkʌp] *n.*

    a medical examination by your doctor or dentist to make sure that there is nothing wrong with your health 体检

13. **mumps** [mʌmps] *n.*

    a disease, especially of children, that causes painful swellings in the neck 腮腺炎

14. **polio** ['pəʊlɪəʊ] *n.*

    an infectious disease that affects the central nervous system and can cause temporary or permanent paralysis 小儿麻痹症

15. **cholesterol** [kə'lestərɔːl] *n.*

    a substance found in blood, fat and most tissues of the body, which can cause heart disease if there is too much of it 胆固醇

16. **diagnostic** [ˌdaɪəg'nɑːstɪk] *n.*

    a distinctive symptom or characteristic 症状

17. **promotion** [prə'məʊʃ(ə)n] *n.*

    activity that encourages people to believe in the value or importance of sth., or that helps sth. to succeed 推广，促进

18. **dramatically** [drə'mætɪklɪ] *adv.*

    in a very dramatic manner 明显地

19. **map** [mæp] *v.*

    to discover or give information about sth., especially the way it is arranged or organized 了解信息，提供信息

20. **potentially** [pə'tenʃəlɪ] *adv.*

    with a possibility of becoming actual 可能地，潜在地

21. **diagnose** [ˌdaɪəg'nəʊs] *v.*

    to say exactly what an illness or the cause of a problem is 诊断（疾病）；判断
    （原因）

22. **disorder** [dɪs'ɔːrdər] *n.*

    an illness that causes a part of the body to stop functioning correctly 紊乱；疾病

23. **viability** [ˌvaɪə'bɪlətɪ] *n.*

    the quality or state of being viable 可行性

24. **launch** [lɔːntʃ] *v.*

    to start an activity, especially an organized one 开始从事；发起

25. **genomic** [dʒiː'nəʊmɪk] *adj.*

    of or relating to genomes 基因组的

26. **initiative** [ɪ'nɪʃətɪv] *n.*

    a new plan for dealing with a particular problem or for achieving a particular
    purpose 新方案；倡议

27. **clinical** ['klɪnɪk(ə)l] *adj.*

    relating to the examination and treatment of patients and their illnesses 临床的

28. **self-medicate** [ˌself 'medɪkeɪt] *v.*

    to administer medication to oneself without medical supervision 自我治疗

29. **nasty** ['næstɪ] *adj.*

    serious 严重的

30. **bump** [bʌmp] *n.*

    a swelling on the body, often caused by a blow 肿块

31. **odds** [ɑːdz] *n.*

    the degree to which sth. is likely to happen 可能性；概率

32. **facilitate** [fə'sɪlɪteɪt] *v.*

    to make an action or a process possible or easier 促进

33. **intervention** [ˌɪntər'venʃ(ə)n] *n.*

    the action or process of intervening 干预

34. **chronic** ['krɑːnɪk] *adj.*

    lasting for a long time or constantly recurring 长期的，慢性的

35. **acute** [ə'kjuːt] *adj.*

having or experiencing a rapid onset and short but severe course 急性的

36. **condition** [kənˈdɪʃ(ə)n] *n.*
    an illness or a medical problem 疾病

Chunk List

Collocations

1. **more... than...** 与其说……倒不如说……
    He's more like a film star than a lifeguard.
    与其说他像个救生员，倒不如说他像个影星。

2. **equate to** 相当于
    We often assume higher price equates to better quality.
    我们通常认为，价格越高质量越好。

3. **up to date** 最新的
    She brought him up to date with what had happened.
    她让他知道了最新的情况。

4. **tailor... to...** 调整，使……适应……
    We can tailor the program to the patient's needs.
    我们可以根据病人的需要调整这个方案。

5. **a good grasp on** 掌握得很好
    He has a good grasp on German grammar.
    他德语语法掌握得很好。

6. **in transition from... to...** 处于由……向……的转变中
    This course is useful for students who are in transition from one training program to another.
    对转换培训项目的学生来说，这一课程是有帮助的。

7. **crucial to** 至关重要
    This game is crucial to our survival.
    这场比赛对我们的生存至关重要。

8. **go away** 消失
    The smell still hasn't gone away.
    气味还没散尽。

9. **at one point** 一度，在某一时刻
    At one point we quarreled over something silly.
    有一次，我们为了一件愚蠢的事争论起来。

Idioms and Proverbs

10. **after the fact** 事后

    On some vital decisions employees were only informed after the fact.

    有一些重大决策雇员只在事后才获悉。

11. **to the forefront** 居于重要地位，引起重视

    This policy brought the disease to the forefront of world attention.

    这项政策使该疾病成为举世瞩目的焦点。

12. **take advantage of** 利用

    She took advantage of the children's absence to tidy their rooms.

    她趁孩子们不在时收拾了他们的房间。

13. **on one's own** 独立地，独自地

    He did it on his own.

    这件事他独立完成了。

14. **be on one's side** 站在某人一边

    I'm definitely on your side in this.

    在这个问题上，我绝对站在你这一边。

(Sub)Technical Chunks

15. **health care** 医疗保健

    Good health care is of primary importance.

    良好的医疗保健是重中之重。

16. **emergency room** 急诊室

    The emergency room was in disorder.

    急诊室里一片混乱。

17. **MBA (Master of Business Administration)** 工商管理学硕士

    An MBA does not guarantee success.

    一个工商管理学硕士学位并不能保证成功。

18. **flu shot** 流感疫苗

    She visited the local clinic for a flu shot.

    她去当地的诊所打了流感疫苗。

19. **blood pressure** 血压

    Your doctor will monitor your blood pressure.

    你的医生会监测你的血压。

20. **genetic testing** 基因检测

    Genetic testing appeals to some people, especially those who are young.

基因检测对一些人很有吸引力，尤其是那些年轻人。

21. **life expectancy** 预期寿命

    A number of social factors influence life expectancy.

    诸多社会因素影响着人的预期寿命。

22. **genetic disorder** 遗传疾病

    His grandchild developed a rare genetic disorder.

    他的孙子得了一种罕见的遗传疾病。

23. **Centers for Disease Control and Prevention** 疾控中心

    The Centers for Disease Control and Prevention estimate that each year, one of every six Americans gets sick from something they eat.

    疾控中心估计，每年每六个美国人中就有一个因为他们所吃的食物而生病。

24. **GP (general practitioner)** 全科医生，普通医师

    You're likely to start by first seeing a GP.

    首先，你可能会去看全科医生。

Sentence Builder

25. **when it comes to...** 当涉及……时

    They are inexperienced when it comes to decorating.

    说到装修，他们没什么经验。

Text B

Heart-health Screenings

1   An important aspect of lowering risk of [1]**cardiovascular disease**, also called [2]**coronary** [3]**artery disease** (CAD), is managing health behaviors and **risk factors**, such as diet quality, **physical activity**, smoking, Body Mass [4]**Index** (BMI), blood pressure, total cholesterol, or **blood** [5]**glucose**. But how do you know which risk factors you have? Your health care professional may conduct or request screening tests during regular visits. Few of us have ideal risk levels on all screening tests. However, if you do have test results that are **less than** ideal, it doesn't mean you're

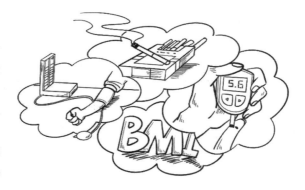

[6]destined to develop a serious cardiovascular disease. On the contrary, it means you're **in a position to** begin changing your health in a positive way.

2   Some measurements such as body weight and blood pressure are taken during routine medical appointments and some cardiovascular screening tests begin at age 20. The frequency of [7]follow-up will depend on your level of risk. You will probably require additional and more frequent testing if you've **been diagnosed with** a cardiovascular condition such as **heart failure** or [8]**atrial** [9]**fibrillation**, or if you have a history of **heart attack**, [10]stroke or other cardiovascular events. Even if you haven't been diagnosed with a condition, your health care professional may want more [11]stringent screening if you already have risk factors or a family history of cardiovascular disease. Here are the key screening tests for [12]monitoring cardiovascular health:

3   Blood pressure is one of the most important screenings because high blood pressure usually has no symptoms so it can't be detected without being measured. High blood pressure greatly increases your risk of heart disease and stroke. If your blood pressure is below 120/80 mm Hg, be sure to get it checked at least once every two years, starting at age 20. If your blood pressure is higher, your doctor may want to check it more often. High blood pressure can be controlled through lifestyle changes and/or [13]medication.

4   You might have a [14]fasting [15]lipoprotein [16]profile (cholesterol) taken every four to six years, starting at age 20. This is a **blood test** that measures total cholesterol, **LDL** (bad) cholesterol and **HDL** (good) cholesterol. You may need to be tested more frequently if your doctor determines that you're at an increased risk for heart disease or stroke. After age 40, your doctor will also want to use an [17]equation to calculate your 10-year risk of experiencing cardiovascular disease or stroke. Like high blood pressure, often cholesterol can be controlled through lifestyle changes and/or medication.

5   Your health care professional may ask for your waist [18]circumference or use your body weight to calculate your Body Mass Index during your routine visit. These measurements may tell you and your physician whether you're at a healthy body weight and [19]composition. Being [20]obese puts you at higher risk for health problems such as heart attack, stroke, atrial fibrillation, [21]congestive heart failure, and more.

6   High blood glucose or "blood sugar" levels put you at greater risk of developing [22]**insulin resistance**, [23]pre-diabetes and **type 2 diabetes**. Untreated diabetes can lead to many serious medical problems including heart disease and stroke. If you're

[24]overweight and you have at least one additional cardiovascular risk factor, your doctor may recommend a blood glucose test. The American Diabetes Association recommends testing for pre-diabetes and risk for future diabetes for all people beginning at age 45. If tests are normal, it is reasonable to repeat testing **at** a minimum of 3-year **intervals**.

7   If you smoke, talk to your doctor at your next health care visit about approaches to help quit. Also discuss your diet and physical activity habits. If there's **room for improvement** in your diet and daily physical activity levels, ask your health care provider to provide helpful suggestions.

8   Below is an [25]overview of heart-health screenings.

Recommended Screenings	How Often
Blood pressure	Each regular health care visit or at least once per year if blood pressure is less than 120/80 mm Hg
Cholesterol ("fasting lipoprotein profile" to measure total, HDL and LDL cholesterol)	Every 4–6 years for normal-risk adults; more often if you have any [26]elevated risk for heart disease and stroke
Weight / Body Mass Index	During your regular health care visit
Waist circumference	As needed to help evaluate cardiovascular risk if your BMI is greater than or equal to 25 kg/m^2
Blood glucose test	At least every 3 years
Discussion of smoking, physical activity, diet	Each regular health care visit

American Heart Association Editorial Staff. 2019. Heart-health screenings. Heart.org.
Retrieved and adapted on August 13, 2022, from Heart.org website.

(730 words)

Notes

1.   (Para. 1) coronary artery disease (CAD)：冠状动脉疾病，又称缺血性心脏病、冠状动脉粥样硬化心脏病、冠状动脉粥样硬化心血管疾病和冠状动脉心脏病，涉及心脏动脉的斑块堆积（动脉粥样硬化），导致流向心肌的血流降低。冠状动脉疾病是最常见的心血管疾病，包含稳定型心绞痛、非稳定型心绞痛、心肌梗死和猝死。

2. (Para. 1) Body Mass Index (BMI)：体质指数，是国际上常用的衡量人体胖瘦程度以及是否健康的一个标准。该指数是由一个人的质量（体重）和身高计算出的一个数值，定义是体重除以身高的平方，以千克/平方米为单位表示。根据各国情况的不同，超重的分界值在22～25之间，肥胖的分界值则在26～31之间。

3. (Para. 1) Few of us have ideal risk levels on all screening tests. However, if you do have test results that are less than ideal, it doesn't mean you're destined to develop a serious cardiovascular disease. 很少有人在所有的筛查项目中都表现出理想的风险水平。然而，如果你的测试结果确实不理想，也并不意味着你注定会患上严重的心血管疾病。

   1）此句中的 do have 表示强调，意为"这种情况确实发生"。

   2）less than ideal：不甚理想，达不到理想的情况。

4. (Para. 2) You will probably require additional and more frequent testing if you've been diagnosed with a cardiovascular condition such as heart failure or atrial fibrillation, or if you have a history of heart attack, stroke or other cardiovascular events. 如果你被诊断患有心力衰竭或心房纤颤等心血管疾病，或者你有心脏病发作、中风或其他心血管疾病的病史，你可能需要额外的、更频繁的检查。

   1）heart failure：心力衰竭，简称心衰，是指由于心脏的收缩功能和（或）舒张功能发生障碍，不能将静脉回心血量充分排出心脏，导致静脉系统血液瘀积，动脉系统血液灌注不足，从而引起心脏循环障碍症候群。此种障碍症候群集中表现为肺瘀血和腔静脉瘀血。心力衰竭并不是一个独立的疾病，而是心脏疾病发展的终末阶段。

   2）atrial fibrillation：心房纤颤，是最常见的心律失常之一，指心房呈无序激动和无效收缩的房性节律，是由心房–主导折返环引起许多小折返环导致的房律紊乱，发病率高，持续时间长，还可引起严重的并发症，如心力衰竭和动脉栓塞。

   3）stroke：中风，又称脑卒中、脑血管意外，一种急性脑血管疾病，是由于脑部血管突然破裂或因血管阻塞导致血液不能流入大脑而引起脑组织损伤的一种疾病，包括缺血性和出血性卒中。中风的发病率、死亡率和致残率都很高，但一直缺乏有效的治疗手段，所以预防是最好的措施。其中，高血压是导致中风的重要可控危险因素。

5. (Para. 2) Even if you haven't been diagnosed with a condition, your health care professional may want more stringent screening if you already have risk factors or a family history of cardiovascular disease. 即使你没有被确诊某种疾病，如果你已经出现风险因素或有心血管疾病家族史，你的医疗保健师也可能会要求你进行更严格的筛查。

6. (Para. 4) You may need to be tested more frequently if your doctor determines that you're at an increased risk for heart disease or stroke. After age 40, your

doctor will also want to use an equation to calculate your 10-year risk of experiencing cardiovascular disease or stroke. 如果你的医生认为你患心脏病或中风的风险在增加，你可能需要更频繁的检查。40 岁以后，你的医生还会用一个公式来计算你 10 年内患心血管疾病或中风的风险。

at an increased risk：风险在增加。

7. (Para. 5) Being obese puts you at higher risk for health problems such as heart attack, stroke, atrial fibrillation, congestive heart failure, and more. 肥胖会增加你心脏病发作、中风、心房纤颤、充血性心力衰竭等疾病的风险。

put sb. at risk：使某人陷入危险。

8. (Para. 6) type 2 diabetes：Ⅱ型糖尿病，旧称非胰岛素依赖型糖尿病或成人发病型糖尿病，是一种慢性代谢疾病，占糖尿病患者的 90% 以上。患者特征为高血糖、相对缺乏胰岛素、胰岛素抵抗等。常见症状有烦渴、频尿、不明原因的体重减轻，可能还包括多食、疲倦或酸痛。高血糖带来的长期并发症包括心脏病、中风、糖尿病视网膜病变，可能导致失明、肾脏衰竭，甚至四肢血流不畅而需要截肢等。

Word List

1. **cardiovascular** [ˌkɑːrdɪəʊ'væskjələr] *adj.*
   connected with the heart and the blood vessels 心血管的

2. **coronary** ['kɔːrənerɪ] *adj.*
   connected with the heart, particularly the arteries that take blood to the heart 冠状动脉的

3. **artery** ['ɑːrtərɪ] *n.*
   any of the tubes that carry blood from the heart to other parts of the body 动脉

4. **index** ['ɪndeks] *n.*
   a system by which changes in the value of sth. and the rate at which it changes can be recorded, measured, or interpreted 指数

5. **glucose** ['gluːkəʊs] *n.*
   a type of sugar that is found in fruit and is easily changed into energy by the human body 葡萄糖

6. **destined** ['destɪnd] *adj.*
   having a future which has been decided or planned at an earlier time, especially by fate 注定的

7. **follow-up** ['fɑːləʊ ʌp] *n.*
   a continuation or repetition of sth. that has already been started or done 后续（行动）；随访

8. **atrial** ['eɪtrɪəl] *adj.*

   of or relating to a cavity or chamber in the body (especially one of the upper chambers of the heart) 心房的

9. **fibrillation** [ˌfɪbrə'leɪʃ(ə)n] *n.*

   a local and uncontrollable twitching of muscle fibers, especially of the heart, not affecting the entire muscle 肌纤维震颤

10. **stroke** [strəʊk] *n.*

    a sudden serious illness when a blood vessel in the brain bursts or is blocked, which can cause death or the loss of the ability to move or to speak clearly 中风

11. **stringent** ['strɪndʒənt] *adj.*

    very strict and that must be obeyed 严格的

12. **monitor** ['mɑːnɪtər] *v.*

    to watch and check sth. over a period of time in order to see how it develops, so that you can make any necessary changes 监测

13. **medication** [ˌmedɪ'keɪʃ(ə)n] *n.*

    a drug or another form of medicine that you take to prevent or to treat an illness 药

14. **fasting** ['fæstɪŋ] *adj.*

    abstaining from food 禁食的

15. **lipoprotein** ['lɪpəprəʊtiːn] *n.*

    a protein that combines with a lipid and carries it to another part of the body in the blood 脂蛋白

16. **profile** ['prəʊfaɪl] *n.*

    an analysis (often in graphical form) representing the extent to which sth. exhibits various characteristics 曲线图

17. **equation** [ɪ'kweɪʒ(ə)n] *n.*

    a statement showing that two amounts or values are equal 方程

18. **circumference** [sər'kʌmfərəns] *n.*

    the length of a line that goes around a circle or any other curved shape 周长

19. **composition** [ˌkɑːmpə'zɪʃ(ə)n] *n.*

    the different parts which sth. is made of 构成

20. **obese** [əʊ'biːs] *adj.*

    very fat, in a way that is not healthy 肥胖的

21. **congestive** [kən'dʒestɪv] *adj.*

   relating to or affected by an abnormal collection of blood or other fluid 充血的

22. **insulin** ['ɪnsəlɪn] *n.*

   a chemical substance produced in the body that controls the amount of sugar in the blood 胰岛素

23. **pre-diabetes** ['prɪˌdaɪə'bɪtɪs] *n.*

   an asymptomatic abnormal state that precedes the development of clinically evident diabetes 糖尿病前期

24. **overweight** [ˌəʊvər'weɪt] *adj.*

   too heavy and fat 超重的

25. **overview** ['əʊvərvjuː] *n.*

   a general description or an outline of sth. 概述

26. **elevated** ['elɪveɪtɪd] *adj.*

   higher than normal 偏高的

Chunk List

Collocations

1. **less than** 不太

   The data was less than ideal.
   数据不太理想。

2. **in a position to do sth.** 处于做某事的适当位置，便于做某事

   I am not in a position to comment.
   我不便发表评论。

3. **be diagnosed with** 被诊断出

   Susan had a mental breakdown and was diagnosed with depression.
   苏珊精神崩溃，被诊断为抑郁症。

4. **at... intervals** 每隔……时间，间或

   The runners started at 5-minute intervals.
   赛跑的人每隔 5 分钟出发一批。

5. **room for improvement** 改进的余地

   There's some room for improvement in your work.
   你的工作还有改进的余地。

(Sub)Technical Chunks

6. **cardiovascular disease** 心血管疾病

Smoking places you at serious risk of cardiovascular disease.

吸烟会大大增加罹患心血管疾病的风险。

7. **coronary artery disease** 冠状动脉疾病，冠心病

Coronary artery disease is the leading cause of death worldwide.

冠状动脉疾病是全球死亡的主要原因。

8. **risk factor** 风险因素

Lack of exercise is a risk factor for heart disease.

缺乏锻炼是导致心脏病的一个因素。

9. **physical activity** 体育活动

Physical activity is an important factor in maintaining fitness.

体育活动是保持健康的一个重要因素。

10. **Body Mass Index** 体重指数

A healthy Body Mass Index is between 18 and 25.

健康的体重指数介于 18 到 25 之间。

11. **blood glucose** 血糖

The levels of blood glucose depend in part on what you eat and when you eat.

血糖水平在一定程度上取决于你吃什么及什么时候吃。

12. **heart failure** 心力衰竭

Her mother died of heart failure.

她母亲死于心力衰竭。

13. **atrial fibrillation** 心房颤动，房颤

Atrial fibrillation can be dangerous, for over time it can cause stroke.

房颤比较危险，因为时间长了它可能导致中风。

14. **heart attack** 心脏病发作

He died of a heart attack brought on by overwork.

他死于劳累过度引起的一次心脏病发作。

15. **blood test** 验血

It may be advisable to have a blood test to put your mind at rest.

验一下血让你自己安心也许是明智的。

16. **LDL (low-density lipoprotein)** 低密度脂蛋白

The new study indicates that the crucial factor is LDL.

这项新的研究表明，低密度脂蛋白才是关键因素。

17. **HDL (high-density lipoprotein)** 高密度脂蛋白

Lack of physical activity may increase LDL and decrease HDL.

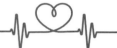

缺乏体育锻炼会增加低密度脂蛋白，降低高密度脂蛋白。

18. **insulin resistance 胰岛素抗性**

Too much insulin is sickening and your body will develop insulin resistance as a result.

太多的胰岛素会引起疾病，你的身体也因此会产生胰岛素抗性。

19. **type 2 diabetes Ⅱ型糖尿病**

Type 2 diabetes is closely linked with obesity.

Ⅱ型糖尿病与肥胖密切相关。

Part 3   Post-reading Exercises

3.1   Read and Answer

3.1.1   Directions: Read Text A in Part 2 and choose the best answers to the following questions.

1. What problem(s) will arise if illnesses are treated after the fact?
   A. Health care issues become more and more serious before they are treated.
   B. Treatment becomes less affordable for patients.
   C. Treatment becomes more expensive for health care providers.
   D. All of the above.

2. By saying "... patient care is more reactive than proactive..." in Paragraph 1, the author implies that _____.
   A. doctors are not very active in treating patients
   B. patients are willing to see doctors
   C. patient care is far from enough
   D. patients tend to get health care after they get sick

3. Which of the following is NOT an advantage of preventive health care?
   A. It addresses health care issues before they get worse.
   B. It is affordable to all patients.
   C. It attempts to deal with an illness before it gets effective treatment.
   D. It can save money for both patients and health care providers.

4. Which of the following is NOT mentioned in the text as an example of widely known preventive care?
   A. Acupuncture.   B. Vaccine.   C. Screening.   D. Test.

5. How do public health programs contribute to preventive care?
    A. They stop people from smoking.
    B. They stress the importance of diet and exercise.
    C. They show people the disadvantages of unhealthy behaviors.
    D. They care about both children and seniors.

6. What do we know about genetic testing according to the text?
    A. It is not likely to predict a patient's future health.
    B. It can't predict the risks of developing common diseases.
    C. It may be helpful in improving the quality of life.
    D. It can be used to cure genetic disorders.

7. From Paragraphs 8 and 9, we can infer that _____.
    A. the success and viability of genetic testing is still in question
    B. EGAPP is not used to test the function of genetic testing
    C. the technology of genetic testing is still being researched
    D. genetic testing has many unsafe and ineffective procedures

8. Why don't people like going to the doctor even when they have some health concerns?
    A. Because they are unwilling to admit that they are sick.
    B. Because their problems are not serious.
    C. Because they can treat all problems by themselves.
    D. Because most illnesses can disappear soon.

9. From the text, we can infer that _____.
    A. health care professionals' experience is more important than learning
    B. all illnesses except the genetic ones are preventable
    C. it is significant for health care professionals to pursue lifelong learning
    D. health care professionals must have a health care MBA degree

10. From which of the following sources is the text most probably selected?
    A. A biology textbook.
    B. A health magazine.
    C. A research paper.
    D. A travel brochure.

3.1.2 Directions: *Read Text B in Part 2 and finish the following exercises. Write T for True, F for False, or NG for Not Given in the brackets before the statements based on the instructions below.*

True   if the statement agrees with the claims of the author;

False	*if the statement contradicts the claims of the author;*
Not Given	*if it is impossible to say what the author thinks about it.*

(   ) **1.** BMI can be used to show a person's health condition to a certain extent.

(   ) **2.** A few people may have ideal risk levels on all screening tests.

(   ) **3.** Body weight and blood pressure are common medical test programs.

(   ) **4.** You need to do more frequent testing if you have been diagnosed with heart failure.

(   ) **5.** Your health care professional won't refer to your family history of cardiovascular disease.

(   ) **6.** It is very important to do screenings of your blood pressure because it's closely related to some diseases.

(   ) **7.** Lifestyle changes or medication can help improve your level of blood pressure and cholesterol.

(   ) **8.** Being obese can definitely lead you to many diseases.

(   ) **9.** Age can influence people's chances of having diabetes.

(   ) **10.** Regular screenings of health behaviors and risk factors are crucial to one's health.

3.2 Guess and Choose

Directions: *Figure out the meanings of the following medical affixes and choose the best answer from the four choices marked A, B, C and D.*

1. arteri, arterio (   )
   A. artery   B. artificial   C. article   D. artist

2. enter, entero (   )
   A. enter   B. intestine   C. entrance   D. entry

3. erythr, erythro (   )
   A. protein   B. nutrient   C. mineral   D. red

4. melan, melano (   )
   A. melon   B. mental   C. black   D. menu

5. therm, thermo (   )
   A. temperature   B. therapy   C. remedy   D. cure

6. pnea (   )
   A. trachea   B. airway   C. nose   D. breath

7. somn, somno (   )
    A. sound　　　　　B. sleep　　　　　C. solid　　　　　D. source

8. pseudo (   )
    A. false　　　　　B. psychology　　　　C. psyche　　　　D. psychiatric

9. scler, sclera, sclerosis (   )
    A. scissors　　　　B. scratch　　　　　C. hardening　　　D. scene

10. angi, angio (   )
    A. blood vessel　　　　　　　　B. blood flow
    C. blood pressure　　　　　　　D. blood clot

3.3 Read and Think

Directions: Read the following medical words built with the medical affixes from Exercise 3.2 and write down their Chinese equivalents in the table below.

Terminology	Chinese Equivalents	Terminology	Chinese Equivalents
arterial		arteriole	
enterovirus		enterocyte	
erythrocyte		erythroblast	
melanoma		melanocyte	
thermal		thermometer	
dyspnea		apnea	
somnia		insomnia	
pseudocyst		pseudogene	
atherosclerosis		arteriosclerosis	
angiography		angioplasty	

3.4 Match and Fill

3.4.1 *Directions: Match the medical terms (a–j) in the box below with their definitions (1–10).*

a. progress	b. checkup	c. polio	d. genetic	e. self-medicate
f. cholesterol	g. stroke	h. obese	i. congestive	j. insulin

(   ) 1.   a general physical examination

(   ) 2.   a chemical substance produced in the body that controls the amount of sugar in the blood

(   ) 3.   to increase in scope or severity, as of a disease taking an unfavorable course

(   ) 4.   a sudden serious illness when a blood vessel in the brain bursts or is blocked, which can cause death or the loss of the ability to move or to speak clearly

(   ) 5.   relating to or affected by an abnormal collection of blood or other fluids

(   ) 6.   an infectious disease that affects the central nervous system and can cause temporary or permanent paralysis

(   ) 7.   having excessive body fat; extremely fat

(   ) 8.   medication of oneself without professional supervision to treat an illness or condition

(   ) 9.   a substance found in blood, fat and most tissues of the body

(   ) 10.   relating to genes, or to the study of genes

3.4.2 Directions: *Make good use of the medical terms you learned from Exercise 3.4.1 and fill in the blanks in the sentences below. Change the form where necessary.*

1.   Remember, DNA is the _____ code for any organism.

2.   Doctor, we both know that people with mental illness often try to _____ with alcohol.

3.   He had a minor _____ in 1987, which left him partly paralyzed.

4.   His illness is likely to _____ into a serious cancer.

5.   It appears to boost the action of _____ and reduce blood sugar.

6.   A person can be overweight without being _____.

7.   Did you have your routine health _____ this year?

8.   In many cases, the cause of _____ heart failure is unknown.

9.   My doctor told me that I need to cut down on eating fried foods in order to improve my _____.

10.   He wore leg braces after he had _____ in childhood.

3.5 Fill and Translate

3.5.1 Directions: Choose the correct medical words from the box below to fill in the gaps (1–10) of the passage concerning fitness and dementia. Change the form where necessary.

develop	onset	stimulation	diagnose	boost
vulnerable	fitness	mechanism	underlying	average

For women, physical fitness in midlife may do more than give the heart a (1) _____; it may also benefit the brain, a new study from Sweden suggests. Researchers found that middle-aged women in Sweden with a high degree of cardiovascular fitness were nearly 90 percent less likely to develop dementia (痴呆) later in life than those who had a moderate fitness level. What's more, if women in the fittest category did develop dementia, these problems—such as trouble with memory and thinking—tended to emerge, on (2) _____, 11 years later than among women in the moderate fitness group. So, the (3) _____ of dementia may have occurred at age 90 in a woman who was considered extremely fit at midlife, compared with age 79 in a moderately fit woman.

The findings suggest that high cardiovascular (4) _____ is associated with a decreased risk of dementia, said lead author Helena Horder, a researcher at the Center for Aging and Health at the University of Gothenburg in Sweden. In other words, good heart health is linked with good brain health, she said. In the study, researchers looked at data from 191 women in Sweden ages 38 to 60. At the start of the study, in 1968, all of the middle-aged women were given an exercise test on a stationary bike in which they cycled until they felt exhausted. After tracking the women for 44 years, the researchers found that those fitness test scores helped predict whether the women would be (5) _____ with dementia later in life. The analysis showed that 32 percent of the women with a low fitness score (6) _____ dementia during the study period, compared with 25 percent of those women with a medium fitness score and 5 percent of the highly fit women. But the highest dementia rates were seen in women who started the exercise test but could not complete it: 45 percent of these women went on to develop dementia. The researchers suspect that some (7) _____ cardiovascular processes—such as high blood pressure—in middle age might have made these women more (8) _____ to dementia decades later.

Previous studies have established a connection between fitness and dementia, but some of them relied on people's self-reported levels of physical activity and did not involve exercise testing. In studies that have shown a link between physical activity and dementia, it's not clear whether the (9) _____ that may be responsible for the brain benefits is an enriched social environment and cognitive (10) _____ or the actual improvement in the fitness level, Horder said.

3.5.2 Directions: *Translate the underlined sentences from the passage above.*

1. Researchers found that middle-aged women in Sweden with a high degree of cardiovascular fitness were nearly 90 percent less likely to develop dementia later in life than those who had a moderate fitness level.

    _____

    _____

2. In other words, good heart health is linked with good brain health, she said.

    _____

    _____

3. At the start of the study, in 1968, all of the middle-aged women were given an exercise test on a stationary bike in which they cycled until they felt exhausted.

    _____

    _____

4. But the highest dementia rates were seen in women who started the exercise test but could not complete it: 45 percent of these women went on to develop dementia.

    _____

    _____

5. Previous studies have established a connection between fitness and dementia, but some of them relied on people's self-reported levels of physical activity and did not involve exercise testing.

    _____

    _____

3.6 Speak and Write

3.6.1 Directions: *Discuss with your group members the phenomenon described in Topic 1 below, and select a representative to report your main ideas to the class.*

Topic 1

"The best physicians start treatment before the outbreak of an illness." (上工治未病)[1] This is a fundamental concept of Chinese health care and medicine, an example of Chinese wisdom in "preparing for rain before a storm" and "guarding against a disaster before it strikes". As an important principle of Chinese medicine, it highly requires a doctor to have a thorough command of pathology and medicine, as well as abilities to anticipate, judge and manage the signs, nature and course of a disease. This ensures early discovery, early prevention and early treatment. Can you give more examples to illustrate this Chinese wisdom?

3.6.2 Directions: *Discuss with your group members the citation below from "Of Studies" written by Francis Bacon and a Chinese proverb in Topic 2 below, and write an essay in about 160 words, concerning self-medication.*

Topic 2

In Francis Bacon's famous essay "Of Studies", he used an analogy "Nay there is no stand or impediment in the wit, but may be wrought out by fit studies: like as diseases of the body may have appropriate exercises. Bowling is good for the stone and reins; shooting for the lungs and breast; gentle walking for the stomach; riding for the head; and the like." There is a similar Chinese proverb " 有病不治，常得中医 "[2], which means that self-treating an illness can usually get a good result. It is similar in meaning to the concept "prolonged suffering from an illness will turn a person into a doctor". It later evolved into sayings like "taking no medicine is better than seeing a mediocre doctor". What is your view on self-medication? Can exercise help treat diseases? Give enough evidence to support your idea.

---

1 《中华思想文化术语》编委会 . 2021. 中华思想文化术语·历史卷 . 北京：外语教学与研究出版社，247.

2 同上：360.

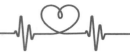

Part 4   **Mini-lecture**

Some Misunderstandings

It's well-known that Chinese learners of English, generally speaking, are superior in receptive skills (i.e. using English to receive information such as reading and listening), but inferior in productive skills (i.e. using English to produce information such as speaking and writing). Even if the students have attained near-native levels of listening and reading skills, they still have much trouble in writing a term paper or effectively expressing a view orally. When asked what impedes their output skills, many students ascribe their productive weakness mainly to a small vocabulary and poor grammar knowledge, followed by other factors such as stage fright, absence of an English-speaking environment, etc. Few would realize that they are not equipped with an adequate reserve of the frequently used idiomatic expressions, namely, chunks.

For decades, both Chinese teachers and learners of English hold the belief that vocabulary and grammar are of paramount importance in learning a language. We all know that words are the smallest unit of a language and grammar is something that combines words into sentences. Therefore, on the one hand, we put heart and soul in enlarging our vocabulary size, and on the other hand, we keep learning grammar rules. We assume that the more words and rules that are at our service, the easier it will be to speak and write good English. Unfortunately, what happens in real life seems to let us down. So, it's time we respectively re-examined vocabulary and grammar, the two most favored elements.

The first is vocabulary. It's worth mentioning that there are about 500,000 words in the language of English. We are actually learning a language which possibly has the largest vocabulary among all languages in the world. Suppose we recite 10 words a day since birth, it'll take us almost 137 years to get the job done, let alone the fact that words change over time, with new words popping up and old ones going out of sight. So, it will surely lead to a problem of cost effectiveness if we blindly absorb as many new single words as possible. Besides, research shows that the average native speaker uses only about 5,000 words to achieve a successful everyday communication. To the majority of Chinese learners, learning 5,000 words is not a daunting task. What may frustrate them is that even though they build that size, they still feel a lot of stresses and strains when it comes to speaking and writing.

The second is grammar. If you believe all the so-called "standard and good" English can be explained by grammar, you're wrong. For example, frequently used phrases such as "day in and day out" "of course" "be in for" "in short", and "from afar" can't be gauged by a grammar yardstick. In addition, it's interesting to see that an average native English speaker has less conscious knowledge of grammar than an average second language learner. But, this "insufficiency" does not prevent them from producing natural and idiomatic English. The knowledge of grammar is not something that matters so much. The thing that does matter is their knowledge of chunks. Native speakers have hundreds of thousands of chunks in their memory and they know what chunks to choose on what occasions.

After re-examining the common belief that the process of learning a language can be simplified as "vocabulary + grammar", we arrive at the conclusion that although there is some truth in it, it overlooks the fact that not all of our language competence has something to do with single words and grammatical rules. The last three decades have seen much interest in the phenomenon of chunks within the second language teaching community. Researchers working in a number of different fields (including computational linguists, lexicographers, discourse analysts, cognitive grammarians, psycholinguists, and language teachers) have emphasized the importance of what is coming to be called "formulaic language" (chunks). Corpus research, particularly, shows that "large parts" of native speakers' vocabulary are organized in terms of strings of words and much language output is not produced in a combing-words-according-to-grammar way, nor much of the standard language can be explained by grammatical rules alone. Though inexplicable, they are used with a high frequency by the native English speakers.

This offers an insight to the advanced English learners such as college students who are eager to yield quality language in their speaking and writing after many years of hard work of building vocabulary and grammar. We have a decision to make: What is worthy of more of our effort in college years? More new single words and grammar rules, or more chunks? When we realize the fact that much of a language consists of chunks which are longer than a single word and much of the real-life communication is operated in terms of the pre-fabricated (pre-made) chunks, we're likely to have some clear ideas.

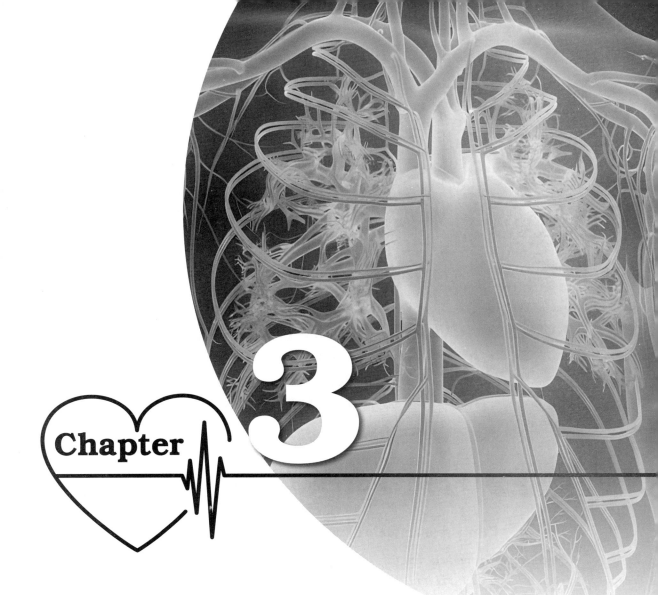

Chapter

3

Chronic Illnesses

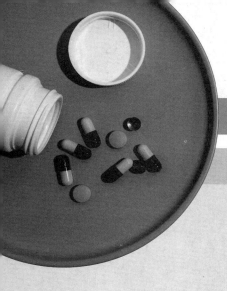

Chapter 3

Chronic Illnesses

Learning Objectives

- to master some basic skills to build medical words with affixes concerning chronic illnesses and to expand accurate usage of amphibious words in both general and medical contexts;

- to improve comprehensive linguistic abilities to discuss chronic illnesses;

- to increase awareness of chronic illnesses and foster a right attitude towards them.

Part 1 **Pre-reading Tasks**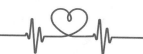

Task 1 **Compare and Contrast**

*Directions: In medical English, **amphibious words**, a term derived from amphibious animals such as frogs and toads that can live both on land and in water, have flexible meanings in both general contexts and medical contexts. Please consult your dictionaries, write down the Chinese equivalents of the amphibious words in the table below, and pay attention to their different meanings used as **general expressions (GE)** and **medical expressions (ME)** respectively. The first one is exemplified for you to follow.*

Amphibious Words	GE	ME
admit	承认；允许；接收	收治，接收入院
case		
clot		
complication		
failure		
murmur		

(Continued)

Amphibious Words	GE	ME
primary		
secondary		
valve		
vessel		

Task 2 Read and Translate

Directions: Please read the following 10 pairs of sentences, and keep an eye on the 10 amphibious words you learned from the table in Task 1, which are interpreted differently as GE and ME. Translate the English sentences into Chinese.

1. She <u>admitted</u> having driven the car without insurance. (GE)

   _____

   _____

   Two crash victims were <u>admitted</u> to the local hospital. (ME)

   _____

   _____

2. You'll probably notice her having difficulty swallowing. If this is the <u>case</u>, give her plenty of liquids. (GE)

   _____

   _____

   Doctors compiled thousands of <u>cases</u> to prove the relationship between smoking and cancer. (ME)

   _____

   _____

3. You silly <u>clot</u>! That's a stupid question. (GE)

   _____

   _____

He needed emergency surgery to remove a blood <u>clot</u> from his brain. (ME)

_____

_____

4. The bad weather added a further <u>complication</u> to our journey. (GE)

_____

_____

Although many carriers have no symptoms, at least one quarter will ultimately suffer some <u>complications</u> from the infection. (ME)

_____

_____

5. But just like the pursuit of perfection is the enemy of progress, so is our fear of <u>failure</u>. (GE)

_____

_____

At least one study showed that women who ate chocolate had a significantly reduced risk of developing heart <u>failure</u>. (ME)

_____

_____

6. He <u>murmured</u> something, and then, food left untouched, went into the sitting room. (GE)

_____

_____

The doctor said James had now developed a heart <u>murmur</u>. (ME)

_____

_____

7. His misunderstanding of language was the <u>primary</u> cause of his other problems. (GE)

_____

_____

The chemotherapy scheme was based on the <u>primary</u> tumor type. (ME)

_____

_____

8. Other consideration is <u>secondary</u> to the major concern of improving efficiency. (GE)

_____

_____

<u>Secondary</u> tumors may be triggered by genetic factors in the internal environment of the organism and factors of the external environment. (ME)

_____

_____

9. Residents heard an enormous bang as a safety <u>valve</u> on the boiler failed. (GE)

_____

_____

One of the effects of the long-lasting infection is the damage to a <u>valve</u> in the heart. (ME)

_____

_____

10. The sailors climbed out of the lifeboat and lifted it slightly up the beach and carelessly glanced at the <u>vessel</u>. (GE)

_____

_____

Severe migraine can be treated with a drug which constricts the blood <u>vessels</u>. (ME)

_____

_____

Task 3 **Lead-in Questions**

Directions: Read the questions below and answer them in details.

1. We use the phrase "chronic illness" to describe an illness that lasts for a long time and difficult to get rid of. Do you know which phrase we use to describe an illness which quickly becomes severe and dangerous?

   _____

   _____

2. Have you or your family members ever been tortured by a chronic illness? If so, please tell us your experience(s).

   _____

   _____

3. A saying goes that "prolonged suffering from an illness will turn a person into a doctor". Please make a comment on the saying.

   _____

   _____

4. What's your view on living with a chronic illness?

   _____

   _____

Part 2　Texts

Text A

A Brighter Holiday After a ¹Pulmonary ²Hypertension Surgery

1　The holiday season is much brighter this year for Laura Floeckhler, 45, from Orlando, Florida. Laura was diagnosed last Christmas with pulmonary hypertension, a type of high blood pressure that affects the arteries in the lungs and the right side of the heart, affecting about 30 in every one million people.

2　Laura's symptoms started earlier in 2014, when the mother of three began experiencing **shortness of breath**. Then her legs and ankles began to [3]swell. As Laura's symptoms worsened, walking became such a struggle that she began filling a [4]cooler with snacks to keep by her bed. "At one point I couldn't walk 10 feet from my bedroom to the kitchen or living room," she says. "Putting on a pair of pants would **knock me out** for the rest of the day."

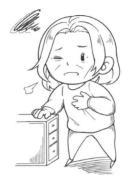

3   On Christmas day 2014, Laura was taken by ambulance to an Orlando community hospital, where she received the [5]diagnosis of pulmonary hypertension. The diagnosis **put her on a path to** Mayo Clinic and regaining her life.

4   Laura was **referred to** Mayo Clinic's Florida campus, where she met Charles Burger, M.D., director of the Clinic Center for Pulmonary Hypertension and [6]**Vascular Diseases**. The center is one of 26 [7]designated centers recognized by the Pulmonary Hypertension Association for its [8]integrative approach to patient care, research and education. With a team of experts, including [9]cardiologists, [10]pulmonologists, interventional [11]radiologists and [12]cardiothoracic [13]surgeons, Mayo is one of the largest centers for treatment of pulmonary hypertension based on patient volumes.

5   "There are five different categories of pulmonary hypertension, so this can be a very difficult disease to diagnose and treat," says Dr. Burger, who [14]**likens** the condition **to** "a [15]kink in a water hose". That causes pressure to build, forcing the right side of the heart to work harder to increase blood flow to the lungs. Eventually, the heart [16]enlarges and fails, Dr. Burger says.

6   Sadly, many patients with pulmonary hypertension are [17]misdiagnosed because a number of conditions have similar symptoms, and the disease has often progressed by the time it is accurately identified. Because of this, some patients require a heart [18]transplant or a heart-lung transplant. "I didn't know how complicated pulmonary hypertension was until I got it and began researching it," says Laura, who on further testing, was found to have a subtype of the condition that causes blood [19]clots in the lungs.

7   Though pulmonary hypertension is a [20]progressive disorder, some patients with Laura's specific condition **are** [21]**eligible for** a complex procedure known as pulmonary [22]thromboendarterectomy, where surgeons [23]scrape the clots from the pulmonary arteries. With the procedure, doctors said Laura could essentially be healed.

8   Getting her active lifestyle back was **within reach**, but Laura feared the worst. Though she hadn't realized it before, Laura learned that another member of her family was diagnosed with the same condition at age 16—but passed away due to [24]complications.

9   Cardiothoracic surgeon Kevin Landolfo, M.D., [25]assured Laura that technology had improved in the past 30 years. Still, thinking about Dr. Landolfo stopping her blood flow and cooling her body to 16–18 **degrees** [26]**Celsius** to remove the clots was frightening. "I was afraid I wouldn't wake up," Laura admits. But she [27]opted to proceed, and in August 2015, [28]underwent the surgery.

10   During the procedure, Dr. Landolfo removed **the majority of** blood clots and scarring from Laura's lungs. "We allowed her lungs to improve, her pressures to go down, and that allows her heart to function in a much more efficient way," says Dr. Landolfo.

11   Almost immediately post-surgery, Laura could **tell the difference**. "Just taking a breath was easier," she recalls. And she was up and walking around the hospital floor the first afternoon.

12   Today, Laura is [29]thrilled to be celebrating the holidays with friends and family, taking in the sights, sounds and smells of the season. She's able to walk freely, is back at work and is looking forward to adventures with her first grandchild.

13   "I love Mayo Clinic and what they did for me," she says. "I feel normal… I feel like I can do it all."

Streed, J. 2015. Holiday season brighter for pulmonary hypertension patient after surgery. Mayo Clinic. Retrieved and adapted on July 16, 2022, from Mayo Clinic website.

(680 words)

Notes

1. (Para. 1) pulmonary hypertension：肺动脉高压，指肺动脉压力升高超过一定界值的一种血流动力学和病理生理状态，可导致右心衰竭。该病可以是一种独立的疾病，也可以是并发症，还可以是综合征。其血流动力学诊断标准为：海平面静息状态下，右心导管检测肺动脉平均压 ≥ 25 mmHg。肺动脉高压是一种常见病、多发病，且致残率和病死率均很高。

2. (Para. 2) As Laura's symptoms worsened, walking became such a struggle that she began filling a cooler with snacks to keep by her bed. 随着劳拉的病症加重，走路已十分费力，她放了一个装满零食的冰箱在床边。

　　1）句中的 worsen 为不及物动词，意为"加重，恶化"。

　　2）such... that...：如此……以致……。that 引导结果状语从句。

3. (Para. 4) The center is one of 26 designated centers recognized by the Pulmonary Hypertension Association for its integrative approach to patient care, research and education. 该治疗中心集护理、研究、教学为一体，是肺动脉高压协会认定的 26 所治疗中心之一。

4. (Para. 7) Though pulmonary hypertension is a progressive disorder, some patients with Laura's specific condition are eligible for a complex procedure known as pulmonary thromboendarterectomy, where surgeons scrape the clots from the pulmonary arteries. 尽管肺动脉高压是一种渐进性疾病，有些与劳拉情况类似的病人符合肺动脉血栓内膜剥脱术的复杂手术条件，可以通过手术剥除动脉血栓。

　　1）progressive disorder：渐进性疾病，指随着时间的推移而恶化和扩散的疾病类型，如渐冻症、渐进性视网膜萎缩、渐进性股骨头坏死等。渐进性疾病可能会造成极其严重的后果，但一部分渐进性疾病可以通过积极治疗而停止或逆转。

　　2）pulmonary thromboendarterectomy：肺动脉血栓内膜剥脱术。其目的是移除肺动脉内血栓及机化内膜，恢复血流灌注和通气血流比例平衡，减轻右室后负荷，避免发生继发性肺血管病。

5. (Para. 9) cardiothoracic surgeon：心胸外科医生，负责心脏外科、胸外科、先天性心脏外科、心肺移植手术等领域的诊疗。此处的 surgeon 指擅长某一类外科手术的医生。

6. (Para. 9) Still, thinking about Dr. Landolfo stopping her blood flow and cooling her body to 16–18 degrees Celsius to remove the clots was frightening. 但想到兰道夫医生在移除血栓时会截断她的血流，把她的身体温度降低到 16—18 摄氏度，她还是感到害怕。

句中的 thinking about... the clots 作主语，其中 stopping her blood flow 和 cooling her body to 16–18 degrees Celsius 是动名词作宾语，指"她"想到的两方面的具体内容。

7. (Para. 10) We allowed her lungs to improve, her pressures to go down, and that allows her heart to function in a much more efficient way... 我们改善了她的肺功能，降低了她的血压，这也使得她的心脏能更高效地运作……

8. (Para. 12) Today, Laura is thrilled to be celebrating the holidays with friends and

family, taking in the sights, sounds and smells of the season. 如今，劳拉正与朋友和家人共度假期，体验当下季节的景色、声音和气息，她为此兴奋不已。

be thrilled to do sth.：对做某事感到兴奋、激动。

9. (Para. 12) She's able to walk freely, is back at work and is looking forward to adventures with her first grandchild. 她能自由行走，回到了工作岗位，并且期待着与她第一个孙辈相见的奇妙经历。

Word List

1. **pulmonary** ['pʌlmənerɪ] *adj.*
   connected with the lungs 肺部的

2. **hypertension** [ˌhaɪpər'tenʃ(ə)n] *n.*
   blood pressure that is higher than normal 高血压

3. **swell** [swel] *v.*
   to become bigger or rounder 肿胀，膨胀

4. **cooler** ['kuːlər] *n.*
   a container or machine which cools things, especially drinks, or keeps them cold 冷藏器

5. **diagnosis** [ˌdaɪəg'nəʊsɪs] *n.*
   the discovery and naming of what is wrong with someone who is ill 诊断

6. **vascular** ['væskjələr] *adj.*
   of or relating to the channels and veins through which fluids pass in the bodies of animals and plants 血管的，维管的

7. **designated** ['dezɪgneɪtɪd] *adj.*
   chosen for a particular job or purpose 指定的；任命的

8. **integrative** ['ɪntɪgreɪtɪv] *adj.*
   combining and coordinating diverse elements into a whole 综合的

9. **cardiologist** [ˌkɑːrdɪ'ɑːlədʒɪst] *n.*
   a doctor who studies and treats heart diseases 心脏病医生，心脏病学家

10. **pulmonologist** [pʌlmə'nɑːlədʒɪst] *n.*
    a specialist in the anatomy, physiology, and pathology of the lungs 胸腔科医师，肺脏学家

11. **radiologist** [ˌreɪdɪ'ɑːlədʒɪst] *n.*
    a doctor who is trained in the branch of medical science that uses X-rays and radioactive substances to treat diseases 放射科医生

12. cardiothoracic [ˌkɑːrdɪəʊθɔːˈræsɪk] *adj.*

of or relating to the heart and the chest 心胸的

13. surgeon [ˈsɜːrdʒən] *n.*

a doctor who is trained to perform the medical operations that involve cutting open a person's body 外科医生

14. liken [ˈlaɪkən] *v.*

to compare one thing or person to another and say they are similar 把……比作

15. kink [kɪŋk] *n.*

a bend or twist in sth. that is usually straight 弯；结

16. enlarge [ɪnˈlɑːrdʒ] *v.*

to become bigger 增大

17. misdiagnose [mɪsˈdaɪəɡnəʊz] *v.*

to diagnose (an illness or problem) wrongly or mistakenly 误诊

18. transplant [trænsˈplænt] *n.*

a medical operation in which a damaged organ, etc. is replaced with one from another person（器官等的）移植

19. clot [klɑːt] *n.*

a lump that is formed when blood dries or becomes thicker（血液的）凝块

20. progressive [prəˈɡresɪv] *adj.*

happening or developing steadily（疾病）渐进性的；稳步的，逐步的

21. eligible [ˈelɪdʒəb(ə)l] *adj.*

having the right to do or obtain sth. 有资格的

22. thromboendarterectomy [ˈθrɑːmbəʊˌendɑːrtəˈrektəmɪ] *n.*

surgical excision of a thrombus and the adjacent arterial lining 血栓动脉内膜切除术

23. scrape [skreɪp] *v.*

to remove sth. from a surface by moving sth. sharp and hard like a knife across it 刮掉，削去

24. complication [ˌkɑːmplɪˈkeɪʃ(ə)n] *n.*

a medical problem that occurs as a result of another illness or disease 并发症

25. assure [əˈʃʊr] *v.*

to tell sb. that sth. is definitely true or is definitely going to happen, especially when they have doubts about it 使……确信，向……保证

26. **Celsius** ['selsɪəs] *n.*

a scale of temperature in which water freezes at 0° and boils at 100° 摄氏（温标）

27. **opt** [ɑːpt] *v.*

to choose to take or not to take a particular course of action 选择

28. **undergo** [ˌʌndər'ɡəʊ] *v.*

to experience sth., especially a change or sth. unpleasant 经历，经受

29. **thrilled** [θrɪld] *adj.*

very excited and pleased 狂喜的

Chunk List

Collocations

1. **knock... out** 使……筋疲力尽

The course completely knocked me out.

这个课程把我累垮了。

2. **put... on a path to** 使……走上……之路

The caring public school teachers put me on a path to success.

这些关心照顾我的公立学校的老师使我走上了成功之路。

3. **refer... to** 将……转交给（以求获得帮助等）

My doctor referred me to a specialist.

我的医生让我去找一位专家（诊治）。

4. **liken... to** 把……比作

Life is often likened to a journey.

（人们）常把人生比作一段旅程。

5. **be eligible for** 有资格

Only those over 70 are eligible for the special payment.

只有 70 岁以上的人才有资格领取这项专款。

6. **the majority of** 大多数

The majority of people interviewed prefer TV to radio.

相比听收音机，大多数接受采访的人更喜欢看电视。

7. **tell the difference** 分辨差别

He didn't seem to be able to tell the difference between right and wrong.

他似乎不能明辨是非。

Idiom and Proverb

8. **within reach** 伸手可及的；在附近

    It saves time in the kitchen to have things you use a lot within reach.

    在厨房里把常用的东西放在手边可以节省时间。

(Sub)Technical Chunks

9. **shortness of breath** 呼吸短促，气短

    Other signs of angina are nausea, sweating, feeling faint, and shortness of breath.

    心绞痛的其他征兆是恶心、出汗、感觉虚弱、晕眩和气短。

10. **vascular disease** 血管性疾病

    Vascular diseases are one of the most serious diseases threatening human health.

    血管性疾病是目前严重威胁人类健康的疾病之一。

11. **degree Celsius** 摄氏度

    It will be a mild night, around nine degrees Celsius.

    晚间天气温和，温度约九摄氏度。

Text B

A Sudden ¹Detour for Heart Transplant

1   In 2015, Yasmin Mullings was ²relishing a fast-paced life. In her role as a county ³prosecutor, she regularly handled complex and challenging cases. Outside of work, she was a ⁴marathon runner, exercise enthusiast, world-traveler and ⁵mentor to middle-school girls. Fit and healthy, Yasmin says medical concerns weren't **on her radar**.

2   That changed dramatically in early 2016. Yasmin returned to running after a short ⁶hiatus, and instead of going her usual 10-plus miles, she couldn't run even one. The incident was the beginning of a medical odyssey that, within six months, took her to Mayo Clinic's Arizona campus, where she ultimately received a heart transplant.

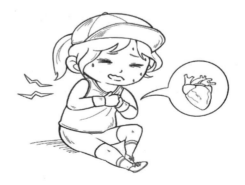

3　In December 2015, Yasmin began the first of three courtroom trials scheduled [7]back-to-back. During that time, she was also training for a marathon. By early February, her [8]grueling schedule had **taken its** [9]**toll**, and she was battling a severe cold. She **took** a few weeks **off** from running, finished the trial, and began to feel better. Yasmin got on her [10]treadmill to restart her marathon training, but before she hit the one-mile mark, she was so short of breath that she had to stop.

4　Her local physicians were [11]stumped, too. Within a month, Yasmin had five medical appointments, with no answers. Meanwhile, her health [12]deteriorated. In early March, she stood up to make an argument in court and briefly **lost** [13]**consciousness**. A trip to the emergency room didn't reveal any clues. She returned home without a solution.

5　Yasmin went back to the local health care clinic the next day and saw a new physician. He suspected something different. He thought her symptoms could be the result of a heart problem and sent Yasmin to see a cardiologist.

6　An [14]echocardiogram and other tests confirmed those [15]suspicions. They revealed that a virus had infected Yasmin's heart, damaging the middle layer of the heart wall, called the [16]myocardium. That condition, known as **viral** [17]**myocarditis**, affected her heart's ability to pump blood and led to heart failure.

7　Heart failure sometimes can be managed with medications. But Yasmin's symptoms continued to get worse despite taking **a variety of** medications. She was in and out of the hospital several times. Then a friend urged her to try a different [18]tactic.

8　In April 2016, Yasmin traveled to Rochester, Minnesota, where she met with John Schirger, M.D., in Mayo Clinic's [19]Division of Cardiovascular Diseases. He told her the tests confirmed the diagnosis of viral myocarditis. He also found that damage from the infection enlarged **the** [20]**chambers of her heart**—a condition called [21]**dilated** [22]**cardiomyopathy**—and that was the [23]underlying cause of Yasmin's heart failure.

9　Yasmin also soon came to realize that her situation was much more serious than she had imagined. Her heart was in severe failure. In the weeks following her first clinic visit, efforts to help it heal didn't work, and she **was admitted to** Mayo Clinic Hospital—Rochester. In early June, Yasmin's care team told her it was time to consider a transplant.

10　"In the first rush of everything, I **was** [24]**bombarded** **with** so much information. But every time the doctors met with me, one of the nurses would stay in the room, too, so I could ask them questions later if I needed to," Yasmin says. "They were there with me, and I never felt like I was on my own," she adds.

11　After **being approved for** a heart transplant and added to the waiting list, Yasmin learned that her wait in Minnesota would likely be 6 to 12 months. With her heart getting worse by the day, her care team feared that she didn't have that long. So they offered another option that she could be [25]transferred to Mayo Clinic's Arizona campus, where her wait for a transplant would likely be shorter. Yasmin quickly agreed. Arrangements were [26]promptly made, and within five days, she was in Arizona.

12　Her care team had been correct in their assessment of the wait time. Yasmin arrived in Arizona on a Thursday. She received her heart transplant the following Wednesday. Recovery went smoothly, and she was back home in St. Paul in less than three months.

13　Yasmin still has regular checkups at Mayo Clinic and requires [27]periodic heart [28]biopsies to make sure her transplanted heart is healthy. Within three months of the transplant, with her care team's encouragement, she was back to running. She's now returned to working full-time, too, although not yet taking courtroom cases. And she's started traveling again.

Sparks, D. Sharing Mayo Clinic: A sudden detour for heart transplant. Mayo Clinic.
Retrieved and adapted on August 19, 2022, from Mayo Clinic website.

(742 words)

Notes

1.　(Para. 1) Outside of work, she was a marathon runner, exercise enthusiast, world-traveler and mentor to middle-school girls. 工作之外，她是马拉松选手，是健身爱好者，是环游世界的旅行家，也是中学女生的辅导教师。
句中并列的"马拉松选手"等四项，表明主人公在工作之外的社会生活中同时兼具多种身份。

2.　(Para. 1) Fit and healthy, Yasmin says medical concerns weren't on her radar. 亚斯敏的身体匀称、健康，她说医疗问题当时根本不在她的考虑范围内。
on one's radar 是一个比喻性的短语，原意为"在某人的雷达扫描范围内"，现多采用其比喻义，表示"在某人的考虑范围内；被某人察觉到"。

3. (Para. 2) a medical odyssey：一场医疗的奇幻之旅。*Odyssey*（《奥德赛》）原为古希腊时期一部著名史诗集的名字，现在多用来指代一段史诗般的征程。

4. (Para. 2) heart transplant：心脏移植术，是将已判定为脑死亡并配型成功的人类心脏完整取出，植入受体胸腔内的同种异体移植手术。受体的自体心脏被移除（称为原位心脏移植）或保留用以支持供体心脏（称为异位心脏移植）。心脏移植手术被视为一种非常规高风险医疗项目，手术的实施主要受科学技术和社会文化两方面的影响，如等待时间长、移植排斥、供体受体选择标准、捐赠流程、伦理、宗教和各地传统文化等因素。

5. (Para. 3) She took a few weeks off from running, finished the trial, and began to feel better. 她休息了几周，没有跑步，完成了庭审案件，感觉身体好转了。
take a few weeks off：休息了几周，放了几周假。

6. (Para. 5) He thought her symptoms could be the result of a heart problem and sent Yasmin to see a cardiologist. 他认为她的症状是由心脏问题引起的，并建议亚斯敏去看心脏科医生。
send sb. to do sth.：派遣某人做某事，指使某人做某事。

7. (Para. 6) viral myocarditis：病毒性心肌炎，指病毒感染引起的心肌局限性或弥漫性的急性或慢性炎症病变，属于感染性心肌疾病。多种病毒可引起心肌炎，其中以引起肠道和上呼吸道感染的病毒最为多见。临床表现取决于病变的广泛程度和部位，轻者可无症状，重者可出现心力衰竭、心源性休克和猝死。目前无特异性治疗方法，治疗主要针对病毒感染和心肌炎症。大多数患者经适当治疗后痊愈，极少数患者在急性期因严重心律失常、急性心力衰竭和 / 或心源性休克死亡。部分患者可演变为扩张型心肌病。

8. (Para. 8) dilated cardiomyopathy：扩张性心肌病，是一种原因未明的原发性心肌疾病，在诊断过程中排除其他特异性原因造成的心脏扩大、心功能不全，根据临床表现及辅助检查即可诊断。其特征为左或右心室或双侧心室扩大，并伴有心室收缩功能减退，伴或不伴充血性心力衰竭。室性或房性心律失常较为多见。病情呈进行性加重，死亡可发生于疾病的任何阶段。

Word List

1. **detour** ['diːtʊr] *n.*
a longer route that you take in order to avoid a problem or to visit a place 绕行的路，迂回路

2. **relish** ['relɪʃ] *v.*
to get great pleasure from sth. 享受，喜爱

3. **prosecutor** ['prɑːsɪkjuːtər] *n.*

a public official who charges sb. officially with a crime and prosecutes them in court 公诉人，检察官

4. **marathon** ['mærəθɑːn] *n.*

   a long running race of about 42 kilometers or 26 miles 马拉松赛跑

5. **mentor** ['mentər] *n.*

   an experienced person who advises and helps sb. with less experience over a period of time 导师；顾问

6. **hiatus** [haɪ'eɪtəs] *n.*

   a pause in which nothing happens, or a gap where sth. is missing 间歇，空隙

7. **back-to-back** [ˌbæk tə 'bæk] *adv.*

   consecutively 连续地

8. **grueling** ['gruːəlɪŋ] *adj.*

   very difficult and tiring, needing great effort for a long time 使人筋疲力尽的

9. **toll** [təʊl] *n.*

   the amount of damage or the number of deaths and injuries that are caused in a particular war, disaster, etc. 伤亡人数；毁坏

10. **treadmill** ['tredmɪl] *n.*

    an exercise machine that has a moving surface that you can walk or run on while remaining in the same place 跑步机

11. **stump** [stʌmp] *v.*

    to ask sb. a question that is too difficult for them to answer or give them a problem that they cannot solve 把……难住，难倒

12. **deteriorate** [dɪ'tɪrɪəreɪt] *v.*

    to become worse 恶化

13. **consciousness** ['kɑːnʃəsnəs] *n.*

    the state of being able to use your senses and mental powers to understand what is happening 清醒，知觉

14. **echocardiogram** [ˌekəʊ'kɑːrdɪəˌgræm] *n.*

    a visual display or record produced using echocardiography 超声心动图

15. **suspicion** [sə'spɪʃ(ə)n] *n.*

    a feeling or belief that sth. is true, even though you have no proof 感觉，看法；猜疑

16. **myocardium** [ˌmaɪə'kɑːrdɪəm] *n.*

    the middle muscular layer of the heart wall 心肌

17. **myocarditis** [ˌmaɪəʊkɑːr'daɪtɪs] *n.*
    inflammation of the heart muscle 心肌炎

18. **tactic** ['tæktɪk] *n.*
    the particular method you use to achieve sth. 策略，手段

19. **division** [dɪ'vɪʒ(ə)n] *n.*
    a large and important unit or section of an organization 部门

20. **chamber** ['tʃeɪmbər] *n.*
    a space in the body, in a plant or in a machine, which is separated from the rest
    腔，室

21. **dilate** [daɪ'leɪt] *v.*
    to become or to make sth. larger, wider or more open（使……）膨胀，（使……）
    扩大

22. **cardiomyopathy** [ˌkɑːrdɪəʊmaɪ'ɑːpəθɪ] *n.*
    chronic disease of the heart muscle 心肌病

23. **underlying** [ˌʌndər'laɪɪŋ] *adj.*
    important in a situation but not always easily noticed or stated clearly 潜在的，
    隐含的

24. **bombard** [bɑːm'bɑːrd] *v.*
    to attack sb. with a lot of questions, criticisms, etc. or by giving them too much
    information 大量提问；大肆抨击；提供过多信息

25. **transfer** [træns'fɜːr] *v.*
    to move sth./sb. from one place to another 转移

26. **promptly** ['prɑːmptlɪ] *adv.*
    immediately 立即，马上

27. **periodic** [ˌpɪrɪ'ɑːdɪk] *adj.*
    happening fairly often and regularly 定期的，周期的

28. **biopsy** ['baɪɑːpsɪ] *n.*
    the removal and examination of tissue from a patient's body, in order to find
    out more about the disease 活组织检查

Chunk List

Collocations

1. **on one's radar** 受某人关注
   The issue of terrorism is definitely on his radar.

恐怖主义问题无疑是他关注的问题。

2. **take... off** 休假，休息
I've decided to take a few days off next week.
我已决定下星期休息几天。

3. **lose consciousness** 失去知觉
When the patient was taken to hospital, he had already lost consciousness.
送到医院时，病人已经昏迷过去了。

4. **a variety of** 各种各样的
The test is used to diagnose a variety of diseases.
此项化验可用于诊断多种疾病。

5. **admit... to (a hospital, an institution, etc.)** 接收……入院，收治……
The mother, who had already lost four children to malaria, was also admitted to hospital for free medical service.
这位被疟疾夺去四个孩子生命的妈妈也被收治入院，接受免费医护。

6. **bombard... with** 大量提问；大肆抨击；提供过多信息
We have been bombarded with letters of complaint.
我们接二连三收到了大批的投诉信件。

7. **be approved for** 获准
Today more than 100 universities have been approved for MBA degrees.
如今，已有 100 多所高校获准授予工商管理硕士学位。

Idiom and Proverb

8. **take its toll** 产生恶果，造成重大损失（或伤亡、灾难等）
The recession is taking its toll on the housing market.
经济衰退使住房市场遭受着重大损失。

(Sub)Technical Chunks

9. **viral myocarditis** 病毒性心肌炎
It can be used for curing viral myocarditis.
它可用于治疗病毒性心肌炎。

10. **the chambers of one's heart** 心腔，心室
Each heartbeat fills the four chambers of her heart with a fresh round of blood.
每次心跳会给她心脏的四个心室供应一股新鲜的血液。

11. **dilated cardiomyopathy** 扩张型心肌病
Dilated cardiomyopathy usually results in congestive heart failure.
扩张型心肌病通常会导致充血性心力衰竭。

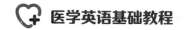

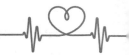

Part 3 　 Post-reading Exercises

3.1 　 Read and Answer

3.1.1　Directions: *Read Text A in Part 2 and choose the best answers to the following questions.*

1. By saying "The holiday season is much brighter this year for Laura Floeckhler…" in Paragraph 1, the author implies that _____.
   A. this year's holiday is not much fun
   B. Laura can better enjoy this holiday without suffering from pulmonary hypertension
   C. Laura's blood clots are reduced
   D. Laura is happy to celebrate the holiday without friends and family

2. Which of the following is true about pulmonary hypertension?
   A. It is a type of low blood pressure.
   B. It affects the arteries in the lungs.
   C. It affects about 30 in every one billion people.
   D. It affects the left side of the heart.

3. Which of the following symptoms did Laura NOT have?
   A. She experienced short breath.
   B. Her legs and ankles began to swell.
   C. She suffered from severe night sweat.
   D. Walking became difficult for her.

4. What is true about Mayo Clinic according to the text?
   A. It doesn't belong to the 26 designated centers recognized by the Pulmonary Hypertension Association.
   B. It has a group of experts, including cardiologists, pulmonologists, interventional radiologists and cardiothoracic surgeons.
   C. It is the second largest center for treatment of pulmonary hypertension.
   D. It only focuses on patient care.

5. Why is it very difficult to diagnose and treat pulmonary hypertension?
   A. Because there are five different categories.
   B. Because many conditions of the disease have similar symptoms.
   C. Because the disease has often progressed by the time it is accurately identified.
   D. All of the above.

6. What did Laura go through during her treatment of pulmonary hypertension?

A. The majority of blood clots and scarring from her lungs were removed.

B. She didn't have any fear at all.

C. She got complications as well.

D. The clots were not removed from her pulmonary arteries.

7. How did Laura feel after the surgery?

A. She still had short breath.

B. She couldn't get up from the bed.

C. She felt much better immediately after the surgery.

D. She couldn't walk around on the first day.

8. The following are all good changes in Laura's life after her pulmonary hypertension is cured EXCEPT that _____.

A. she is happily enjoying her life

B. she is able to walk freely

C. she needs some time to have a rest away from work

D. she is anticipating her first grandchild

9. This text is most likely found in a book of _____.

A. entertainment

B. novel

C. clinical cases

D. fairy tales

10. What is the main idea of this text?

A. An introduction to pulmonary hypertension.

B. The symptoms of pulmonary hypertension.

C. An introduction to Mayo Clinic.

D. The story of Laura who finally recovered from pulmonary hypertension.

3.1.2 **Directions:** *Read Text B in Part 2 and finish the following exercises. Write T for True, F for False, or NG for Not Given in the brackets before the statements based on the instructions below.*

True	*if the statement agrees with the claims of the author;*
False	*if the statement contradicts the claims of the author;*
Not Given	*if it is impossible to say what the author thinks about it.*

(   ) **1.** Before 2016, Yasmin didn't have any medical concerns.

(   ) **2.** Yasmin was a sports lover in 2015.

(　　) 3. An incident happened to Yasmin which didn't stop her from running 10-plus miles.

(　　) 4. Busy schedules had no influence on Yasmin's health conditions at all.

(　　) 5. No one knew what was wrong with Yasmin's health at first, even her local physicians.

(　　) 6. Medications were effective in dealing with Yasmin's condition.

(　　) 7. Yasmin's heart failure was caused by viral myocarditis.

(　　) 8. Yasmin was transferred to Mayo Clinic's Arizona campus because she could get a transplant quicker there.

(　　) 9. Yasmin's transplanted heart is healthy now and she no longer returns to her courtroom cases.

(　　) 10. Life was gradually back to normal after the heart transplant for Yasmin.

3.2 Guess and Choose

Directions: Figure out the meanings of the following medical affixes and choose the best answer from the four choices marked A, B, C and D.

1. cardi, cardio (　　)
   A. heart　　　　B. cargo　　　　C. cardinal　　　　D. carbon

2. pulmon, pulmono (　　)
   A. chest　　　　B. neck　　　　C. lungs　　　　D. arm

3. pneum, pneuma, pneumat, pneumato (　　)
   A. energy　　　　　　　　　　B. lungs and breath
   C. mouth　　　　　　　　　　D. air and fluid

4. thorac, thorax (　　)
   A. throat　　　　B. thorn　　　　C. throne　　　　D. chest

5. thromb, thrombo (　　)
   A. clot　　　　B. thumb　　　　C. trunk　　　　D. threat

6. ectomy (　　)
   A. ecology　　　　B. eclipse　　　　C. resection　　　　D. ecstatic

7. my, myo (　　)
   A. muscle　　　　B. marrow　　　　C. bone　　　　D. mouth

8. itis (　　)
   A. irritation　　　　B. allergy　　　　C. influenza　　　　D. inflammation

9. vas, vaso, vasculo (   )
   A. blood tube   B. vase   C. blood flow   D. vehicle

10. hyper (   )
    A. low   B. high   C. beneath   D. under

3.3 Read and Think

Directions: Read the following medical words built with the medical affixes from Exercise 3.2 and write down their Chinese equivalents in the table below.

Terminology	Chinese Equivalents	Terminology	Chinese Equivalents
echo**cardio**gram		**cardio**logist	
pulmonary		**pulmon**ologist	
pneumonia		**pneumon**ic	
cardio**thorac**ic		**thorax**	
thrombectomy		**thromb**osis	
append**ectomy**		gast**rectomy**	
myocardium		**myo**cardial	
myocard**itis**		bronch**itis**	
vascular		**vas**ectomy	
hypertension		**hyper**active	

3.4 Match and Fill

3.4.1 Directions: Match the medical terms (a–j) in the box below with their definitions (1–10).

a. artery	b. radiologist	c. surgeon	d. misdiagnose
e. transplant	f. complication	g. deteriorate	h. echocardiogram
i. medication	j. biopsy		

(   ) 1. a secondary disease, an accident, or a negative reaction occurring during the course of an illness and usually aggravating the illness

(   ) 2. a vessel through which the blood passes away from the heart to various parts of the body

(   ) 3. a non-invasive ultrasound test that shows an image of the inside of the heart

(   ) 4.   a physician trained in the use of radioactive substances, X-rays, and other imaging techniques

(   ) 5.   to grow worse in function or condition

(   ) 6.   a doctor who treats disease, injury, and deformity by operation or manipulation

(   ) 7.   a drug or other substance used to treat disease or injury; a medicine

(   ) 8.   to make an incorrect diagnosis of (a particular illness)

(   ) 9.   the removal and examination of a sample of tissue from a living body for diagnostic purposes

(   ) 10.   to transfer (tissue, a body structure, or an organ) from one body to another body or from one part of the body to another part

3.4.2 Directions: *Make good use of the medical terms you learned from Exercise 3.4.1 and fill in the blanks in the sentences below. Change the form where necessary.*

1.   The heart _____ will take place as soon as a suitable donor can be found.

2.   _____ provides information about the size and shape of your heart and how well your heart chambers and valves are functioning.

3.   He had an operation last year to widen a heart _____.

4.   Blindness is a common _____ of diabetes.

5.   A(n) _____ should read a CAT head scan within 45 minutes of the patient's arrival.

6.   Clinical assessment and imaging studies are helpful but a tissue _____ is often required.

7.   He is reputed to be the best heart _____ in the country.

8.   It is probable that the _____ will suppress the symptom without treating the condition.

9.   In many cases, doctors _____ patients or give them the wrong treatment or not enough treatment.

10.   However, in the last 20 years of his life, his health began to _____ and he was miserable.

3.5   Fill and Translate

3.5.1 Directions: *Choose the correct medical words from the box below to fill in the gaps*

(1–10) of the passage concerning excessive blood clotting. Change the form where necessary.

artery	complication	fail	medication	misdiagnose
myocardium	pulmonologist	clot	surgery	underlying

When you get a cut or wound, your body forms blood clots, a thickened mass of blood tissue, to help stop the bleeding. After bleeding has stopped and healing has occurred, the body should break down and remove the (1) _____. But sometimes they form too easily or don't dissolve properly and travel through the body limiting or blocking blood flow. This is called excessive blood clotting or hypercoagulation, and can be very dangerous. In a case of excessive blood clotting, these clots can form in, or travel to, the (2) _____ or veins in the brain, heart, kidneys, lungs and limbs, which in turn can cause heart attack, stroke, damage to the body's organs or even death.

Many factors can cause excessive blood clotting, including certain diseases and conditions, genetic mutations (突变) and (3) _____. These causes fall into two categories: acquired and genetic. Acquired means that excessive blood clotting was triggered by another disease or condition. The genetic, or inherited, source of excessive blood clotting is less common and is usually due to genetic defects. These defects usually occur in the proteins needed for blood clotting and can also occur with the substances that delay or dissolve blood clots. Acquired and genetic sources of excessive blood clotting are not related but a person can have both.

There are many possible (4) _____ of blood clots. For example, a stroke can occur if a blood clot causes blood flow to your brain to be restricted. If blood flow is cut off for more than a few minutes, the cells in your brain start to die. A stroke can cause lasting brain damage, long-term disability, paralysis, or death.

A blood clot in a coronary artery can lead to a heart attack. A heart attack occurs if blood flow to a section of heart muscle becomes blocked. If blood flow isn't restored quickly, the (5) _____ becomes damaged from lack of oxygen and begins to die. This heart damage may not be obvious, or it may deteriorate or cause long-lasting problems such as heart (6) _____ or arrhythmias (心律不齐).

A blood clot can also be a(n) (7) _____ cause to kidney failure, where kidneys can no longer remove fluids and waste from your body.

If a blood clot travels from a deep vein in the body to the lungs, it's called a(n)

(8) _____ obstruction (栓塞), which is a serious condition that can damage your lungs and other organs and cause low oxygen levels in your blood. It can often be (9) _____ as a stroke, heart attack or pneumonia because of the symptoms similar to other conditions.

With medicines and ongoing care, many people who have excessive blood clotting can successfully manage it. Your doctor may advise (10) _____ if your blood clot is very large and is causing severe tissue injury. While surgery is not the only kind of treatment for a blood clot, most people with blood clots are treated with medicines called blood thinners.

3.5.2 Directions: *Translate the underlined sentences from the passage above.*

1. When you get a cut or wound, your body forms blood clots, a thickened mass of blood tissue, to help stop the bleeding.

    _____

    _____

2. Acquired means that excessive blood clotting was triggered by another disease or condition.

    _____

    _____

3. These defects usually occur in the proteins needed for blood clotting and can also occur with the substances that delay or dissolve blood clots.

    _____

    _____

4. A stroke can cause lasting brain damage, long-term disability, paralysis, or death.

    _____

    _____

5. A heart attack occurs if blood flow to a section of heart muscle becomes blocked.

    _____

    _____

3.6 Speak and Write

3.6.1 ***Directions:*** *Discuss with your group members the phenomenon described in Topic 1 below, and select a representative to report your main ideas to the class.*

Topic 1

Asthma is the most common chronic disease in children and the leading cause of pediatric hospitalization worldwide. The incidence and prevalence of childhood asthma increased markedly during the 20th century, especially in developing countries. In China, the prevalence of asthma among urban children has increased dramatically from 1.5% to 6.8% over the past decade. It is suggested that environmental factors are likely responsible for the increase in the prevalence of asthma. The rapid increasing quantity of vehicles in recent years has led to combined classical industrial and modern traffic air pollution in China. What do you think of the role air pollution played in childhood asthma?

3.6.2 ***Directions:*** *Discuss with your group members the phenomenon described in Topic 2 below, and write an essay in about 160 words, entitled "My View on Hypertension Prevalence in China".*

Topic 2

High blood pressure is often referred to as the "silent killer" since it may show no symptoms but can put you at an increased risk for the heart attack, heart failure, and stroke, among other things. The prevalence of hypertension in China has been increasing in the last decades. According to a recent survey, a total of 26.6% of Chinese adults had hypertension, and a significantly greater number of men were hypertensive than women, The age-specific prevalence of hypertension was 13% among young people (aged 20–44), 36.7% among the middle-aged (45–64), and 56.5% among the elderly people (aged 65 and above) respectively. In economically developed regions, the prevalence of hypertension was significantly higher among rural residents than among urban residents. Among hypertensive patients, 45% were aware of their condition, 36.2% were treated, and 11.1% were adequately controlled. Some argue that hypertension is a by-product of economic prosperity, do you agree? What can we do to improve hypertension awareness, control, and treatment in China?

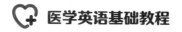

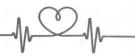

Part 4 · Mini-lecture

The Benefits of Learning Chunks

Learning chunks has been viewed as an essential element in achieving native-like production and as the key to the general language acquisition process. Research findings suggest that the mental lexicon does not consist solely of words, but also large chunks of language. Therefore, there has been a significant trend that chunks should transcend single words and be the focus of vocabulary teaching and learning, especially to the advanced learners of English. "You shall know a word by the company it keeps", to quote a saying from the famous British linguist Firth. Here, "keep somebody company" is a chunk, too.

Abundant research indicates that the ability to identify, memorize and internalize (i.e. make it part of the way you think and behave) chunks is a short-cut to the improvement of language competence. The benefits of learning chunks can be summarized as follows:

- Learning chunks promotes native-like fluency. It helps the learners to cope with the demands of real-time language comprehension and production while maintaining fluency, because it's more likely to achieve native-like fluency when the speakers don't construct each sentence from the scratch. Let's take clothe-making as an example to illustrate this view. Suppose you go to your tailor and place an order for a shirt in the morning. You ask it to be done before dinner on the same day. Because you are a regular customer, the tailor happens to have something ready-made for you in advance, say, a collar, front, back and sleeves. So this time, all the tailor has to do is put these pieces together and he can meet the deadline without much effort. But, what if the tailor has nothing ready-made beforehand? What if he has to make the shirt stich by stich? Maybe, he will miss the deadline. This alludes to the process of making a sentence. If you have a large bank of pre-made chunks at your hand, you can avoid building every sentence word by word, namely from the scratch. It saves you much time to construct a sentence chunk by chunk, and thus guarantees fluency.

- Leaning chunks promotes native-like selection. It helps the learners to produce natural language in contrast to expressions that are grammatical but are judged to be "unidiomatic". The capacity to sound idiomatic is to speak a second language in a way a native speaker of that language would. Even though many learners achieve native-like fluency, they fail to achieve native-like selection. In other words, they can produce language at a rate not particularly different from that produced by native speakers, but they still sound "foreign" and "odd" because their choice of language makes it clear that they are operating on a different system. Chinese English such as "When the tiger is not in the mountain, the monkey becomes the king" （山中无老虎，猴子称大王）, "living level" （生活水准）, "common friend" （共同的朋友）, are a sure result of an insufficient knowledge of chunks. On the contrary, if you have a good command of those frequently used idiomatic expressions, you will not find it a daunting task to produce idiomatic translations for the above: "When the cat's away, the mice will play" "living standard" "mutual friend". Native-speaker proficiency requires one to have an enormous repertoire of chunks that has to be accessible; hence an appropriate selection can be made. World famous linguist Skehan pointed out in 1998 that foreign language leaners who restrict themselves to item(word)-and-rule approaches to language will be forever marked as non-members of the speech community they aspire to.

- Learning chunks promotes creation. While memorized chunks can provide a quick route into fluent and native-like speech, learners will ultimately need to tailor their production to new situations and to express ideas effectively and freely. Linguists and researchers have concluded that it is precisely through the learning of ready-made chunks that mastery of the creative and abstract patterns of language is best achieved. For example, a journalist wants to write an article about Rome, the capital city of Italy. To make it eye-catching and impressive, he entitled the article "There's No Place like Rome", which is actually a reference to the household saying "There's no place like home". With this, the journalist departs from the normal pattern of a language and becomes a creative language user. Therefore, a good command of a considerable number of chunks such as collocations, idioms, famous sayings and maxims, key sentence patterns, ready-made sentences of much practical use, and so on and so forth, is essential for the creative element to take effect and yield speeches that are original, acceptable and natural to a native ear. Besides, it should be pointed out that an excellent grasp of chunks does not only help you to yield creative use of language, but also help understand and appreciate it when a skilful writer or speaker departs from the normal patterns of a language.

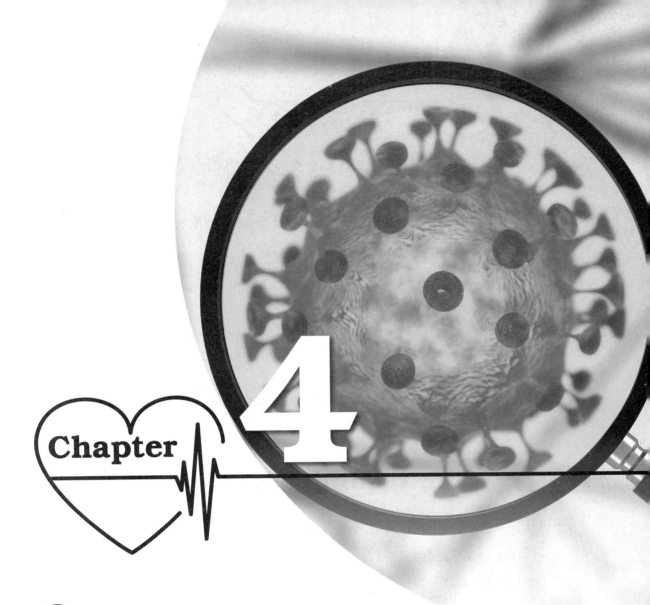

Chapter **4**

Cancers

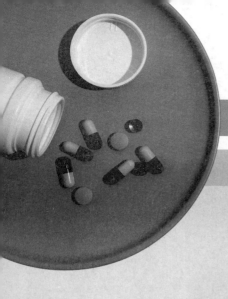

Chapter 4
Cancers

Learning Objectives

- to master some basic skills to build medical words with affixes concerning tumors and cancers and to expand accurate usage of amphibious words in both general and medical contexts;

- to improve comprehensive linguistic abilities to discuss some life-threatening diseases such as cancers;

- to increase awareness of cancers and foster a right attitude towards them.

Part 1   Pre-reading Tasks

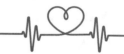

Task 1   Compare and Contrast

*Directions: In medical English, **amphibious words**, a term derived from amphibious animals such as frogs and toads that can live both on land and in water, have flexible meanings in both general contexts and medical contexts. Please consult your dictionaries, write down the Chinese equivalents of the amphibious words in the table below, and pay attention to their different meanings used as **general expressions (GE)** and **medical expressions (ME)** respectively. The first one is exemplified for you to follow.*

Amphibious Words	GE	ME
agent	代理人	药剂
deliver		
gum		
mass		
persistent		
prescribe		

(Continued)

Amphibious Words	GE	ME
progress		
positive		
negative		
resistance		

Task 2 **Read and Translate**

Directions: Please read the following 10 pairs of sentences, and keep an eye on the 10 amphibious words you learned from the table in Task 1, which are interpreted differently as GE and ME. Translate the English sentences into Chinese.

1. As an <u>agent</u>, you may have an inside track when good deals become available. (GE)

   _____

   _____

   After the patient took contrast <u>agent</u>, her image quality had marked improvement. (ME)

   _____

   _____

2. She is due to <u>deliver</u> a lecture on genetic engineering. (GE)

   _____

   _____

   Her husband had to <u>deliver</u> the baby himself on the way to hospital. (ME)

   _____

   _____

3. I've tried everything from herbal cigarettes to chewing <u>gum</u>. (GE)

   _____

   _____

The toothbrush gently removes plaque without damaging the gums. (ME)

_____

_____

4. She portrays herself as both a queen and mother to the masses. (GE)

_____

_____

Ultrasonography reported a big gas-filled mass in the lower abdomen. (ME)

_____

_____

5. It would be much more satisfactory if new ideas were the just reward for hard work and persistent effort. (GE)

_____

_____

Symptoms of the illness include a high temperature and a persistent dry cough. (ME)

_____

_____

6. The teaching syllabus prescribes precisely which books should be studied. (GE)

_____

_____

Our doctor diagnosed a throat infection and prescribed antibiotic and junior aspirin. (ME)

_____

_____

7. There is no straightforward equivalence between economic progress and social well-being. (GE)

_____

_____

Their brains are scanned so that researchers can monitor the <u>progress</u> of the disease. (ME)

_____

_____

8. Overseas investment has had a <u>positive</u> effect on exports. (GE)

_____

_____

The athlete tested <u>positive</u> for steroids and then was dismissed from the final match. (ME)

_____

_____

9. When asked for your views about your current job, on no account must you be <u>negative</u> about it. (GE)

_____

_____

Most important, your <u>negative</u> test result shows you were not infected. (ME)

_____

_____

10. <u>Resistance</u> to change has nearly destroyed the industry. (GE)

_____

_____

Antibiotic <u>resistance</u> is one of the world's most pressing public health problems. (ME)

_____

_____

Task 3 Lead-in Questions

Directions: Read the questions below and answer them in details.

1. Do you believe there's a connection between what we eat every day and the development of a cancer? Why or why not?

   _____

   _____

2. Do you think a healthy lifestyle is essential to reduce the incidence of cancers? Why or why not?

   _____

   _____

3. Is stress management important in preventing people from developing cancers? Are you strong in stress management? Why or why not?

   _____

   _____

4. How do you evaluate the importance of doing regular exercise in inhibiting life-threatening diseases?

   _____

   _____

Part 2　Texts

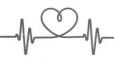

Text A

You Have to Have Faith to Survive

1　As a professional mental health ¹counselor, I have years of experience helping others work through issues in their own lives. I know the importance of staying positive during difficult times and not letting negative thoughts ²**cloud your mind**, especially when important decisions need to be made. But it wasn't until I went through a hardship of my own that I realized the true importance of that ³mindset.

2　It was during a trip to visit my son in Texas that the pain began. It became so

[4]unbearable that I was forced to go to the emergency room. The doctors there told me I had a [5]perforated [6]ulcer that would need to be operated on immediately. It was a very scary experience, but the idea of having cancer never entered my mind. After the initial surgery, however, a similar pain returned.

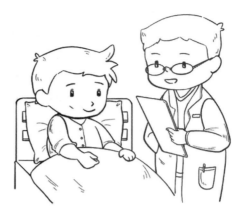

3   In September 2015, a [7]recurrence [8]prompted my doctor to schedule an [9]endoscopy. I tried not to worry, I tried to **put into practice** the positive thinking I discuss with my clients, but I found that was **easier said than done**. My **heart sank** as the doctor **delivered the news**; I had stage 2 stomach cancer. At first, it was hard to accept the news. My mind began to race and questions and doubts clouded my mind. Why was this happening to me? How would I **get through** this? Would I **make it**?

4   As soon as I found out I had cancer, I knew immediately that I wanted to be treated at a cancer center. I made my appointment at Fox Chase, Pennsylvania (PA) and from the first moment I entered the building, all of the negative thoughts, all of my anxieties, began to **fade away**. Everyone was so positive and encouraging and I left my initial [10]consultation with a [11]surgical [12]oncologist feeling hopeful.

5   When I first met with my doctor, my family and I were full of questions. He patiently answered **each and every** question, and I [13]**plucked up** enough **courage** step by step. After initial testing, it was determined that I would need two months of [14]chemotherapy followed by surgery to remove the [15]tumor in my stomach. [16]Prepping for the surgery was [17]nerve-wracking, but I found the entire staff of doctors, nurses, techs, and receptionists extremely friendly and supportive. I also found my doctor to be a very devoted and experienced doctor. Through help from my family, support from the staff at Fox Chase, and continued prayer, I went into my surgery feeling positive about the outcome.

6   The morning of March 8, 2016 was one I will never forget. **Nervous as I was**, sitting in the surgical waiting room, I had an [18]undercurrent of confidence. Of course, my surgical oncologist did an amazing job with the surgery, removing the ulcer and cancerous mass completely, leaving only a small [19]incision behind. I had little post-surgery pain and spent five days as an [20]inpatient. During that time, I was, again, impressed by the level of kindness and ²¹compassion displayed by the staff at Fox Chase, especially when, following the procedure, I underwent additional rounds of chemotherapy, at a hospital near my home. The Fox Chase staff worked with staff members at my local hospital to ensure I was given the best care possible. After months of chemotherapy, on October 10, 2016, I was finally cancer free.

7   Your life with cancer is definitely different; **there is no doubt about** that. But difference doesn't necessarily mean worse. For me, I have learned to **be** more ²²**attuned to** my body. I watch what I eat, and when my stomach bothers me, I **reach out to** my medical team. I am much more cautious than before. I feel more ²³empathic at work. As a counselor it is my job to help others work through issues in their lives. Because of this cancer journey, I feel I am that much more qualified to help my clients.

8   My family, friends, and coworkers were all ²⁴pivotal to the positive attitude I maintained through my journey. Now, time spent with them is even more precious. I even regularly ²⁵skype with my grandson who lives in Germany.

9   I would not have got through this without my doctor and all of the staff at Fox Chase. ²⁶Gloomy as it may seem, always surround yourself with people to help you get through the tough times. You have to have faith; you have to believe you will be one of the people who survive.

Pyle, P. 2022. Patient story. Fox Chase. Retrieved and adapted on August 15, 2022, from Fox Chase website.

(747 words)

Notes

1.   (Para. 1) But it wasn't until I went through a hardship of my own that I realized the true importance of that mindset. 直到我亲身经历了一番痛楚艰辛，才真正意识到保持乐观心态有多重要。
It was not until... that... 为强调句。

2.   (Para. 4) Fox Chase (Fox Chase Cancer Center)：福克斯·蔡司癌症中心，坐落于宾夕法尼亚州的费城，始建于 1904 年，是美国最早的癌症医院之一。其所属的医疗中心是一所教学医院性质的综合医院。福克斯·蔡司癌症中心的医学家在癌症预防、诊断、治疗和癌症存活方面取得了突破，并在各自领域获得了最高奖项，包括两项诺贝尔奖。

3.   (Para. 4) Everyone was so positive and encouraging and I left my initial consultation

with a surgical oncologist feeling hopeful. 每个人都如此地积极乐观，鼓舞人心。
在一位外科肿瘤专家初诊后，我看到了希望。

此句中的 feeling hopeful 为状语性分词结构。此类结构有助于简化行文，为主句
提供时间、因果、方式、背景、动机等信息。

4. (Para. 6) Nervous as I was, sitting in the surgical waiting room, I had an
    undercurrent of confidence. 在手术等候室，尽管我很是紧张，但心底涌起一股信心。
    句首的 Nervous as I was 为倒装结构。由 as/though 引导的让步状语从句用倒装语
    序时，把从句的表语或状语等放在 as/though 前面，例如：
    Young as she was, she stood up bravely against her uncle.

5. (Para. 6) inpatient：住院病人。比较：outpatient 意为 "门诊病人"。

6. (Para. 8) skype：打网络通话。Skype 为全球免费的语音沟通软件，具备即时通讯
    所需的多种功能，如视频聊天、多人语音会议、多人聊天、传送文件、文字聊天等。
    它可以高清晰地与其他用户语音对话，也可以拨打国内、国际电话。2013 年 3 月，
    微软在全球范围内关闭了即时通讯软件 MSN，由 Skype 取而代之。

7. (Para. 9) I would not have got through this without my doctor and all of the staff
    at Fox Chase. 如果没有主治医生和福克斯·蔡司的所有员工，我挺不过这一关。
    句中的 would not have got through 为虚拟语气。

Word List

1. **counselor** ['kaʊnsələr] *n.*
    a person who has been trained to advise people with problems, especially
    personal problems 顾问

2. **cloud** [klaʊd] *v.*
    to make (a matter or mental process) unclear or uncertain; to confuse 使……模糊；
    使……迷惑

3. **mindset** ['maɪndset] *n.*
    a set of attitudes or fixed ideas that sb. has and that are often difficult to change
    观念模式，思维倾向

4. **unbearable** [ʌn'berəb(ə)l] *adj.*
    too painful, annoying or unpleasant to deal with or accept 难以忍受的

5. **perforate** ['pɜːrfəreɪt] *v.*
    to make a hole or holes through sth. 打孔，穿孔

6. **ulcer** ['ʌlsər] *n.*
    a sore area on the outside of the body or on the surface of an organ inside the

body which is painful and may bleed or produce a poisonous substance 溃疡

7. **recurrence** [rɪ'kɜːrəns] *n.*

happening again (especially at regular intervals) 重现，复发

8. **prompt** [prɑːmpt] *v.*

to make sb. decide to do sth. 促使，导致

9. **endoscopy** [en'dɑːskəpɪ] *n.*

a medical operation in which an endoscope is put into a person's body so that the parts inside can be seen 内窥镜检查

10. **consultation** [ˌkɑːns(ə)l'teɪʃ(ə)n] *n.*

a meeting with an expert, especially a doctor, to get advice or treatment 就诊；咨询会

11. **surgical** ['sɜːrdʒɪk(ə)l] *adj.*

used in or connected with surgery 外科的

12. **oncologist** [ɑːn'kɑːlədʒɪst] *n.*

a specialist in the scientific study of and treatment of tumors in the body 肿瘤医师，肿瘤学家

13. **pluck** [plʌk] *v.*

to make a sharp pull or twitch 拽，拉

14. **chemotherapy** [ˌkiːməʊ'θerəpɪ] *n.*

the treatment of disease, especially cancer, with the use of chemical substances 化学治疗

15. **tumor** ['tuːmər] *n.*

a mass of cells growing in or on a part of the body where they should not, usually causing medical problems 肿瘤

16. **prep** [prep] *v.*

to prepare (sth.) 准备

17. **nerve-wracking** ['nɜːrvˌrækɪŋ] *adj.*

making you feel very nervous and worried 令人焦虑不安的

18. **undercurrent** ['ʌndərkɜːrənt] *n.*

a feeling, especially a negative one, that is hidden but whose effects are felt 潜在的情绪

19. **incision** [ɪn'sɪʒ(ə)n] *n.*

a sharp cut made in sth., particularly during a medical operation 切口

20. **inpatient** ['ɪnˌpeɪʃ(ə)nt] *n.*

    a person who stays in a hospital while receiving treatment 住院病人

21. **compassion** [kəm'pæʃ(ə)n] *n.*

    a strong feeling of sympathy for people who are suffering and a desire to help them 同情，怜悯

22. **attuned** [ə'tuːnd] *adj.*

    familiar with sb./sth. so that you can understand or recognize them and act in an appropriate way 熟悉的，习惯的

23. **empathic** [em'pæθɪk] *adj.*

    showing empathy or ready comprehension of others' states 感同身受的

24. **pivotal** ['pɪvət(ə)l] *adj.*

    of great importance because other things depend on it 关键性的

25. **skype** [skaɪp] *v.*

    to communicate, or communicate with, using Skype (a computer program that you can use to make voice calls or video calls on the Internet)（用Skype软件进行）网络通话

26. **gloomy** ['gluːmɪ] *adj.*

    sad and without hope 忧郁的，无望的

Chunk List

Collocations

1. **cloud one's mind** 使某人思绪不清

    Doubts were beginning to cloud my mind.

    种种疑问开始使我的思路变模糊了。

2. **put... into practice** 实施，落实

    The difference between successful and unsuccessful people is that successful people put into practice the things they learn.

    成功者和失败者的区别在于，成功者将他们所学的东西付诸实践。

3. **easier said than done** 说来容易做起来难

    Avoiding mosquito bites is easier said than done.

    防蚊叮咬说来容易做起来难。

4. **heart sinks** 情绪低落

    My heart sank when I saw so much work.

    当我看到有那么多活时，心情顿时沮丧。

5. **deliver the news** 宣布消息

The mayor delivered the unwelcome news that city employees may have to take unpaid time off.

市长宣布了人们不想听到的消息——所有城市雇员可能停薪休假。

6. **get through** 熬过

It is hard to see how people will get through the winter.

很难想象人们将怎样熬过这个冬天。

7. **fade away** 逐渐消逝

Hopes of reaching an agreement seem to be fading away.

达成协议的希望看来已逐渐渺茫。

8. **each and every** 每一个

Offering advice on each and every problem will undermine her feeling of being adult.

每个问题都为她提出忠告会逐渐削弱她的成年意识。

9. **be attuned to** 熟悉，习惯

She wasn't yet attuned to her baby's needs.

她还没有熟悉她宝宝的需要。

10. **reach out to** 愿意倾听

So far, his administration has failed to reach out to Republicans.

他的政府至今没有表现出愿意倾听共和党意见的姿态。

Idioms and Proverbs

11. **make it** 幸免于难，渡过难关

The doctors think he's going to make it.

医生们认为他能挺过去。

12. **pluck up (the) courage** 鼓起勇气

I finally plucked up (the) courage to ask her for a date.

我终于鼓起勇气约她出去。

Sentence Builders

13. **Nervous as I was...** 尽管我很紧张……

Nervous as I was, I finished the task successfully.

尽管我很紧张，我还是成功地完成了任务。

14. **There is no doubt about...** ……是毫无疑问的，毫无疑问……

He's made some great movies. There's no doubt about it.

他拍了一些非常出色的影片。这一点是毫无疑问的。

Text B

A Difficult Journey as an AML Patient

1 When I initially contacted the general ¹practitioner (GP), I informed her that I had ²tonsilitis symptoms. She ³dismissed the tonsilitis as a "viral illness" and I was told to **ride** it **out** for a few days and if it got any worse, she would ⁴prescribe me ⁵antibiotics for three days' time. I **ended up** taking the antibiotics as it did get worse, **to the point** where I couldn't speak; the pain was incredible. On the Monday I was ⁶vomiting

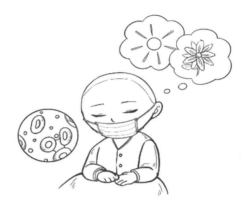

blood which I thought was maybe ⁷gastrointestinal (GI) bleeding. As a nurse myself, I rang the emergency call to explain that I had some signs of tonsilitis and fresh blood followed by ⁸coffee-ground vomit.

2 I attended my local **accident and emergency (A&E) department** on the advice of the GP. After waiting for about three hours, I was ⁹triaged by the nurse; my **heart rate** was high and blood pressure quite low. She was **keeping her eye on** me. Then it was my turn to be reviewed by the A&E ¹⁰consultant. Full history was taken, I explained about my throat being sore and coughing up the blood, so a full examination was completed, blood was taken, and he took my pulse ¹¹manually. The recording was so high on the ¹²cardiac monitor, ranging from 140–160 bpm. Initially, we both thought it was because I was ¹³dehydrated and a bag of ¹⁴intravenous (IV) fluids and IV antibiotics would **do the trick** and I would be on my way.

3 My blood came back and the consultant came in to tell me that my ¹⁵potassium was low on the blood gas and gave me some IV fluids with potassium. He didn't mention anything about my full **blood count** (FBC) at this point, and then repeated my blood test. A few hours later, the consultant came back with my blood test results saying to me "I have some bad news... You have a white cell count greater than 200 and ¹⁶platelets of 14. As a nurse working in ¹⁷hematology, you must know what that means." Yes, I did know what that meant but I made him tell me in his words not mine. That's when he told me, "it looks like you have acute ¹⁸leukemia". The next hour or two were a ¹⁹blur; all I can remember is that I rang my parents and other family members to tell them the doctors think I have leukemia and I was hoping that it wasn't. I informed my friends and colleagues of the diagnosis, some of them crying.

4 I was then seen by the hematologist **on call** from Southport hospital. He was asking me lots of questions about the symptoms of leukemia—any [20]bruising? Any abnormal bleeding? Bleeding from the [21]gums? I didn't have any of these. When my potassium [22]stabilized, my hematologist confirmed that I had AML and suggested [23]leukapheresis to remove them. Even though I had the knowledge about the signs of leukemia, I didn't spot the signs as the symptoms are so vague!

5 Following this in my head I thought to myself "It's here; it needs to go." I signed the [24]**consent form** for treatment and then waiting for what felt like forever to get my **PICC** line inserted. When that was in, I had some platelets and then my first cycle of chemotherapy that evening. As the days went on, I did get severely [25]unwell; I was even seen by a doctor from **intensive care** due to having multiple infections, even struggling to breathe. It was madness how I went from having no symptoms of having AML to being very [26]poorly within days of being admitted.

6 Being a nurse doesn't mean you will have **a narrow escape**. I now have a better understanding of what it actually feels like to be **on the receiving end of** having chemotherapy and the **side effects** patients actually go through **first hand**. Post four cycles of chemotherapy, I underwent a stem cell transplant to ensure full [27]remission and stop the cancer from coming back. Thankfully my lovely older brother is my [28]donor.

7 There is a long recovery ahead. **Fight or flight kicks in**; for me it was fight. It is scary when hair starts to fall out but remember it's only hair, and it will grow back. It's a difficult journey but you must be honest with yourself. Not every day is sunshine and daisies, but having a positive mental attitude has helped me through the horrible six months and to think about what's ahead. Some days stay gold forever.

Lawrenson, A. 2022. Untitled. Leukaemiacare. Retrieved and adapted on July 30, 2022, from Leukaemiacare website.

(756 words)

Notes

1. (Title) AML (acute myelocytic leukemia): 急性髓细胞白血病，是最常见的白血病

类型之一。根据累及细胞序列的不同，白血病可以分为急性髓细胞白血病和急性淋巴细胞白血病两大类。临床中，急性髓细胞白血病可分为 M0—M7，一共八种。发病机制是骨髓中异常的原始细胞及偏原始的幼稚细胞（白血病细胞）大量增殖并抑制正常造血功能，浸润肝、脾、淋巴结、皮肤黏膜等器官。其临床表现主要有贫血、出血、感染、肝脾淋巴结肿大、骨骼关节疼痛等症状。

2. (Para. 1) general practitioner (GP)：全科医生，在美国也被称为家庭医生，是综合程度较高的医学人才，主要为社区家庭提供基本、连续、综合的医疗卫生保健服务。全科医生是接触患者的第一道门槛，他们对病人的疾病或伤势进行初步诊断，决定基础的诊疗方案，负责健康维护、诊疗、转科、协调及随访，在美国的医疗系统中起着很重要的作用。

3. (Para. 1) coffee-ground vomit：呕吐咖啡渣样物，是指上消化道出血引起的呕吐物呈棕褐色，类似咖啡渣样的表现。这是因为血液在胃内停留的时间较长，红细胞被破坏，经胃酸作用后，呕吐物便呈棕褐色。

4. (Para. 3) full blood count (FBC)：全血细胞计数，是一项筛选性检查，众多的疾病在诊断时都需要用到这项检查。通过这项检查，医生可以观察到血细胞的增多、减少、被破坏等情况，从而了解炎症、过敏、血凝等情况，这对于疾病的诊断与治疗有着极其重要的作用。

5. (Para. 4) 注意区分 symptoms 与 signs。symptoms 意为"症状"，是指患者主观感受到的不适，比如发烧、头晕；signs 意为"体征"，是医生依靠自己的感官或者医疗器械发现的患者的病理生理变化。

6. (Para. 5) PICC (peripherally inserted central catheter)：经外周静脉置入中心静脉导管。它由外周静脉（贵要静脉、肘正中静脉、头静脉）穿刺插管，其尖端位于上腔静脉下 1/3，用于为患者提供中长期的静脉输液治疗。导管材料为硅胶，柔软、弹性好，对血管刺激性小，可长期留置，为危重患者的抢救治疗、监测及胃肠外营养治疗、肿瘤化疗提供了有效途径。

7. (Para. 5) intensive care：重症监护。intensive care unit (ICU) 意为"重症监护室"，它把危重病人集中起来，在人力、物力和技术上给予最佳保障，以期得到良好的救治效果。ICU 设有中心监护站，直接观察所有监护的病床。ICU 的设备必须配有床边监护仪、中心监护仪、多功能呼吸治疗机、麻醉机、心电图机、除颤仪、起搏器、输液泵、微量注射器、处于备用状态的吸氧装置、气管插管及气管切开等所需急救医疗设备。

8. (Para. 6) stem cell transplant：干细胞移植。干细胞是骨髓最早制造出、最原始且未特化的细胞，具有发展成许多不同细胞类型的潜力。干细胞移植治疗是把健康的干细胞移植到患者体内，以达到修复或替换受损细胞或组织，进而治愈的目的。干细胞移植治疗范围很广，一般能治疗神经系统疾病、免疫系统疾病以及其他的一些内外科疾病。对于影响骨髓和血液的癌症，如白血病、淋巴瘤、骨髓瘤、神经胚细胞瘤或其他血液疾病，干细胞治疗可直接对抗它们，当然也可帮助缓解症状。

Word List

1. **practitioner** [præk'tɪʃ(ə)nər] *n.*
   a person who works in a profession, especially medicine or law 从业人员

2. **tonsilitis** [ˌtɑːnsə'laɪtɪs] *n.*
   an infection of the tonsils in which they become swollen and sore 扁桃体炎

3. **dismiss** [dɪs'mɪs] *v.*
   to decide that sb./sth. is not important and not worth thinking or talking about 不予考虑，摒弃

4. **prescribe** [prɪ'skraɪb] *v.*
   to tell sb. to take a particular medicine or have a particular treatment 给……开（药），让……采用（疗法）

5. **antibiotics** [ˌæntɪbaɪ'ɑːtɪks] *n.*
   medical drugs used to kill bacteria and treat infections 抗生素

6. **vomit** ['vɑːmɪt] *v. & n.*
   to bring food from the stomach back out through the mouth; food from the stomach brought back out through the mouth 呕吐；呕吐物

7. **gastrointestinal** [ˌgæstrəʊɪn'testɪn(ə)l] *adj.*
   of or relating to the stomach and intestines 胃肠的

8. **coffee-ground** ['kɔːfɪˌgraʊnd] *adj.*
   resembling the dregs remaining after brewing coffee 咖啡渣状的

9. **triage** ['triːɑːʒ] *v.*
   to decide how seriously ill/sick or injured a person is, so that the most serious cases can be treated first 鉴别分类患者，分诊

10. **consultant** [kən'sʌltənt] *n.*
    a hospital doctor of the highest rank who is a specialist in a particular area of medicine 高级顾问医师

11. **manually** ['mænjʊəlɪ] *adv.*
    by hand rather than automatically or using electricity, etc. 手动地

12. **cardiac** ['kɑːrdɪæk] *adj.*
    connected with the heart or heart disease 心脏的，心脏病的

13. **dehydrate** [diː'haɪdreɪt] *v.*

to make a person's body lose too much water 使（身体等）脱水

14. **intravenous** [ˌɪntrəˈviːnəs] *adj.*
    going into a vein 静脉输入的

15. **potassium** [pəˈtæsɪəm] *n.*
    a chemical element in combination with other minerals in the body that are important in body processes and play an essential role in maintenance of the acid-base and water balance in the body 钾

16. **platelet** [ˈpleɪtlət] *n.*
    a very small part of a cell in the blood, shaped like a disc, which helps to clot the blood from a cut or wound 血小板

17. **hematology** [ˌhiːməˈtɑːlədʒɪ] *n.*
    the scientific study of the blood and its diseases 血液学

18. **leukemia** [luːˈkiːmɪə] *n.*
    a serious disease in which too many white blood cells are produced, causing weakness and sometimes death 白血病

19. **blur** [blɜːr] *n.*
    sth. that you cannot remember clearly 模糊的记忆

20. **bruising** [ˈbruːzɪŋ] *n.*
    a blue, brown or purple mark that appears on the skin after sb. has fallen, been hit, etc. 瘀伤

21. **gum** [ɡʌm] *n.*
    either of the firm areas of flesh in the mouth to which the teeth are attached 牙龈

22. **stabilize** [ˈsteɪbəlaɪz] *v.*
    to become firm, steady and unlikely to change; to make sth. stable（使……）稳定

23. **leukapheresis** [ˈluːkəfrɪsɪs] *n.*
    a medical procedure that separates and removes excessive leukocytes from a patient's blood 白细胞去除术

24. **consent** [kənˈsent] *n.*
    permission to do sth., especially given by sb. in authority 同意

25. **unwell** [ʌnˈwel] *adj.*
    sick 不舒服的，生病的

26. **poorly** [ˈpʊrlɪ] *adj.*
    sick 不舒服的，生病的

27. **remission** [rɪ'mɪʃ(ə)n] *n.*

a state or period during which a serious illness improves for a time and the patient seems to get better 缓解，缓解期

28. **donor** ['dəʊnər] *n.*

a person who gives blood or a body organ to be used by doctors in medical treatment 献血者，器官捐献者

Chunk List

Collocations

1. **ride out** 安然渡过

   Most large companies should be able to ride out the recession.
   大多数大公司应该能安然渡过经济衰退期。

2. **end up doing sth.** 最终成为，到头来

   I ended up doing all the work myself.
   结果所有的活儿都是我一个人干了。

3. **to the point** 达到某种程度，近乎

   He was rude to the point of being aggressive.
   他粗鲁到蛮不讲理的地步。

4. **a narrow escape** 死里逃生，侥幸脱险

   I hear you had a very narrow escape on the bridge.
   我听说你在桥上侥幸脱险。

5. **on the receiving end of** 成为（不愉快事件的）承受方

   She found herself on the receiving end of a great deal of criticism.
   她发现自己遭到众多的批评。

6. **first hand** 直接地

   We've been through Germany and seen first hand what's happening there.
   我们曾走遍德国，目睹了那里发生的事。

7. **fight or flight** 战斗还是逃跑

   I guess this is a case of fight or flight.
   我猜想这是该决定战斗还是逃跑的时候了。

8. **kick in** 开始生效或见效

   Reforms will kick in later this year.
   改革将于今年下半年开始见效。

Idioms and Proverbs

9. **keep an eye on** 留神，照看

   We've asked the neighbors to keep an eye on the house for us while we are away.

   我们已经请邻居在我们离开时帮忙照看一下房子。

10. **do the trick** 奏效，达到目的

    I don't know what it was that did the trick, but I am definitely feeling much better.

    我不知道是什么起了作用，但是我确实觉得好多了。

11. **on call**（尤指紧急情况下）随叫随到

    I'll be on call the night of the party.

    在聚会的晚上我将随时听凭召唤。

(Sub)Technical Chunks

12. **AML (acute myelocytic leukemia)** 急性髓细胞白血病

    She was diagnosed with AML.

    她被诊断出患有急性髓细胞白血病。

13. **accident and emergency (A & E) department** 急诊室

    She began vomiting blood and was rushed to the accident and emergency department.

    她开始吐血，于是被急忙送到急诊室。

14. **heart rate** 心率

    When we exercise, our heart rate increases.

    当我们锻炼时，心率会加速。

15. **blood count** 血细胞总数，血细胞计数

    We do a blood count to ensure that all is well.

    我们进行了血细胞计数，确保一切正常。

16. **consent form** 同意书

    Before an operation the patient will be asked to sign a consent form.

    手术前，患者将被要求在同意书上签字。

17. **PICC (peripherally inserted central catheter)** 经外周静脉置入中心静脉导管

    The study seeks to explore the value of PICC in preterm infants.

    此项研究试图探讨经外周静脉置入中心静脉导管在早产儿中的应用价值。

18. **intensive care** 特别护理，重症监护

    She needed intensive care for several days.

    她需要几天的重症特别护理。

19. **side effect**（药物的）副作用

Depression is a side effect of many medications.

抑郁是很多药物都会产生的一种副作用。

Part 3 Post-reading Exercises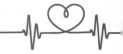

3.1 Read and Answer

3.1.1 Directions: *Read Text A in Part 2 and choose the best answers to the following questions.*

1. What does "that mindset" refer to in the last line of Paragraph 1?

   A. Helping others solve problems in their lives.

   B. Staying positive during difficult times.

   C. Having negative thoughts.

   D. Making important decisions.

2. Which of the following feelings did the author NOT experience upon knowing she had cancer?

   A. Worry.　　　　B. Doubt.　　　　C. Anxiety.　　　　D. Calmness.

3. Which of the following is NOT a factor contributing to the author's courage to fight against cancer?

   A. Everyone was positive and encouraging at Fox Chase.

   B. The author's condition was not that serious.

   C. The doctor was patient to answer every question.

   D. The entire staff at Fox Chase was very friendly and supportive.

4. Which of the following is true according to the text?

   A. The author was very confident when waiting for the surgery.

   B. The author got no pain after the surgery.

   C. The author's ulcer and cancerous mass were completely removed.

   D. The author only had chemotherapy at Fox Chase.

5. How was the author's post-cancer life?

   A. She was more used to her body.

   B. She paid attention to what she ate.

   C. She became more cautious about her health.

   D. All of the above.

6. Who are NOT mentioned as a big support for the author during her cancer journey?

   A. Family.

   B. Friends.

   C. Clients.

   D. Colleagues.

7. What's the author's overall attitude towards her whole cancer journey?

   A. Positive.

   B. Negative.

   C. Resentful.

   D. Gloomy.

8. This text would most likely be used to _____.

   A. encourage people with cancer to have faith to survive

   B. introduce a mental health counselor's life

   C. advise people on how to stay positive

   D. tell people how to support a cancer patient

9. From the text, we can infer that _____.

   A. a mental health counselor won't be negative easily

   B. it is easier said than done

   C. the author got much help, kindness and compassion at Fox Chase

   D. people around cancer patients have a big influence on them

10. What is the main idea of this text?

   A. The author's life as a mental health counselor.

   B. How the author survived cancer.

   C. The importance of support for cancer patients.

   D. The author's post-cancer life.

3.1.2 ***Directions:*** *Read Text B in Part 2 and finish the following exercises. Write T for True, F for False, or NG for Not Given in the brackets before the statements based on the instructions below.*

> *True*   *if the statement agrees with the claims of the author;*
>
> *False*   *if the statement contradicts the claims of the author;*
>
> *Not Given*   *if it is impossible to say what the author thinks about it.*

(   ) 1. The author's tonsilitis symptoms got worse and worse so that she even couldn't speak.

(   ) 2. Antibiotics can be used to treat tonsilitis.

(　　) 3. As a nurse, the author knew exactly why she was vomiting blood.

(　　) 4. Nothing was told to the A&E consultant before the author took a full examination.

(　　) 5. After two blood tests, the author was confirmed to have acute leukemia.

(　　) 6. The author didn't tell anyone about the bad news of her diagnosis.

(　　) 7. Symptoms of leukemia may include bruising, abnormal bleeding, bleeding from the gums, etc.

(　　) 8. The author could better understand what patients went through after getting sick herself.

(　　) 9. The author got much support and compassion from other patients.

(　　) 10. Staying positive helped the author a lot in fighting against AML.

3.2 Guess and Choose

Directions: Figure out the meanings of the following medical affixes and choose the best answer from the four choices marked A, B, C and D.

1. onco (　　)
    A. only   B. cancer   C. one   D. single

2. oma (　　)
    A. tumor   B. oasis   C. oat   D. oath

3. carcin, carcino (　　)
    A. carrot   B. carbon   C. carry   D. cancer

4. gastr, gastro (　　)
    A. belly   B. bowel   C. stomach   D. intestine

5. hemo, haema, hemat, hemato (　　)
    A. blood   B. uria   C. gland   D. fluid

6. leuk, leuko, leuco (　　)
    A. red   B. orange   C. black   D. white

7. emia (　　)
    A. blood vessel   B. blood cell   C. blood condition   D. bleeding

8. myel, myelo (　　)
    A. muscle   B. marrow   C. bone   D. joint

9. chemo, chemi (　　)
    A. chemical   B. physical   C. mental   D. spiritual

10. scopy (　　)

    A. visual examination　　　　　B. physical check-up

    C. microscope　　　　　　　　D. macroscope

3.3　Read and Think

Directions: *Read the following medical words built with the medical affixes from Exercise 3.2 and write down their Chinese equivalents in the table below.*

Terminology	Chinese Equivalents	Terminology	Chinese Equivalents
oncologist		**onco**logy	
fibr**oma**		lymph**oma**	
carcinoma		**carcino**gen	
gastrologist		**gastro**scopy	
hematology		**hemo**globin	
leukocyte		**leuka**pheresis	
leuk**emia**		an**emia**	
myeloma		**mye**litis	
chemotherapy		**chemi**cals	
endo**scopy**		colono**scopy**	

3.4　Match and Fill

3.4.1　Directions: *Match the medical terms (a–j) in the box below with their definitions (1–10).*

a. ulcer	b. surgery	c. tumor	d. incision	e. inpatient
f. prescribe	g. antibiotics	h. vomit	i. leukemia	j. hematologist

(　　) 1.　a cut into a body tissue or organ, especially one made during surgery

(　　) 2.　to eject matter from the stomach through the mouth

(　　) 3.　a sore area on the outside or inside of your body which is very painful and may bleed or produce a poisonous substance

(　　) 4.　a person staying in a hospital, at least overnight, for treatment

(　　) 5.　an acute or chronic disease in humans and other warm-blooded animals characterized by an abnormal increase in the number of white blood cells in the tissues and often in the blood

(　　) 6.　the treatment of diseases, injuries and deformities by physical, manual or instrumental interventions

(　　) 7.　a medical specialist who treats diseases and disorders of the blood and blood-forming organs

(　　) 8.　to order the use of (a medicine or other treatment)

(　　) 9.　a mass of cells in your body that grow in a way that is not normal

(　　) 10.　medical drugs used to kill bacteria and treat infections

3.4.2　Directions: *Make good use of the medical terms you learned from Exercise 3.4.1 and fill in the blanks in the sentences below. Change the form where necessary.*

1.　He needed a(n) _____ to cure a troublesome back injury.

2.　I got a throat infection last week and had to go to the hospital to get some _____ as I really wasn't getting any better.

3.　Please do not directly paste it to skin of the _____ and the wound.

4.　Tommy lost his appetite and began to _____ shortly after he ate the street food.

5.　Generally outpatient costs are not covered and only 60% of _____ hospital bills are compensated.

6.　Both won the Nobel Prize and had _____ because of radioactivity.

7.　Unfortunately, the girl he truly fell in love with had a brain _____ that put her into a coma.

8.　Two Chinese scientists, material expert Shi Changxu and _____ Wang Zhenyi won China's top science award.

9.　Ask your doctor to _____ a medicine to help prevent allergies.

10.　To prevent an infection in your _____, keep it dry and clean.

3.5　Fill and Translate

3.5.1　Directions: *Choose the correct medical words from the box below to fill in the gaps (1–10) of the passage concerning cancers. Change the form where necessary.*

chemotherapy	ulcer	gastrointestinal	cancerous	tissue
diagnose	secondary	tumor	mass	lymph

In the most basic terms, cancer refers to cells that grow out of control and invade other tissues. Cells may become (1) _____ due to the accumulation of defects, or mutations in their DNA. Certain inherited genetic defects and infections can increase the risk of cancer. Most of the time, cells are able to detect and repair DNA damage. If a cell is severely damaged and cannot repair itself, it usually undergoes so-called programmed cell death. Cancer occurs when damaged cells grow, divide, and spread abnormally instead of self-destructing as they should.

A tumor is an abnormal (2) _____ of cells. Tumors can either be benign (non-cancerous) or malignant (cancerous). Benign tumors grow locally and do not spread. As a result, benign (3) _____ are not considered cancer. They can still be dangerous, especially if they press against vital organs like the brain. Malignant tumors have the ability to spread and invade other tissues.

Metastasis is the process whereby cancer cells break free from a malignant tumor and travel to and invade other (4) _____ in the body. Cancer cells metastasize to other sites via the (5) _____ system and the bloodstream. Cancer cells from the original—or primary tumor can travel to other sites such as the lungs, bones, liver, brain, and other areas. These metastatic tumors are "secondary cancers" because they arise from the primary tumor.

Certain genes control the life cycle—the growth, function, division, and death of a cell. When these genes are damaged, the balance between normal cell growth and death is lost. Cancer cells are caused by DNA damage and out-of-control cell growth. Cancer may be caused by environmental exposure. Sunlight can cause cancer through ultraviolet radiation. Some microbes (微生物) are known to increase cancer risks. These include bacteria like H. pylori, which causes stomach (6) _____ and has been linked to (7) _____ cancer. Viral infections have also been linked to cancer. Lifestyle choices can lead to cancer as well. Eating a poor diet, inactivity, obesity, heavy alcohol use, smoking, and exposure to chemicals and toxins are all associated with greater cancer risk.

Medical treatment with (8) _____, radiation, targeted treatments or immunosuppressive drugs used to decrease the spread of cancer throughout the body can also cause damage to healthy cells. Some "(9) _____ cancers", completely separate from the initial cancer, have been known to occur following aggressive cancer treatments; however, researchers are producing drugs that cause less damage to healthy cells, for example, targeted therapy. Cancers that are aggressive or (10) _____ at a later stage may be more difficult to treat, and can even be life-threatening.

3.5.2 Directions: *Translate the underlined sentences from the passage above.*

1. Certain inherited genetic defects and infections can increase the risk of cancer.

   _____

   _____

2. Cancer occurs when damaged cells grow, divide, and spread abnormally instead of self-destructing as they should.

   _____

   _____

3. Malignant tumors have the ability to spread and invade other tissues.

   _____

   _____

4. These metastatic tumors are "secondary cancers" because they arise from the primary tumor.

   _____

   _____

5. Eating a poor diet, inactivity, obesity, heavy alcohol use, smoking, and exposure to chemicals and toxins are all associated with greater cancer risk.

   _____

   _____

3.6 Speak and Write

3.6.1 Directions: *Discuss with your group members the phenomenon described in Topic 1 below, and select a representative to report your main ideas to the class.*

Topic 1

Cancer patients can feel depression and anxiety any time after a cancer diagnosis. Psychological distress, such as chronic depression and anxiety, is a typical problem. In the context of cancer patients, prevalence rates of psychological distress are four times higher than that in the general population and often elicit worse outcomes. Studies have confirmed the links between psychological distress and cancer progression. In a way, chronic stress promotes tumor growth. What are your suggestions for cancer patients and their families?

3.6.2 **Directions:** *Discuss with your group members the phenomenon described in Topic 2 below, and write an essay in about 160 words, entitled "My View on Presymptomatic Testing for Cancers".*

Topic 2

Breast cancer is by far the most common cancer among women. It is estimated that about one tenth of annual breast-cancer-related deaths can be traced to a germ-line defect. Of the 10% who have an inherited susceptibility to breast cancer, one half can be traced to mutations of the BRCA1 gene, a big gene with numerous variants. It appears that the BRCA2 gene accounts for most of the other half of the germ-line defects. The testing for BRCA1/2, the genetic predisposition for breast cancer, helps to discover a mutated gene before any signs of illness.

Presymptomatic testing for perilous, incurable diseases will certainly do a lot of good, but it will also give rise to problems which are ethical in nature. Certain ethical principles have to be respected, for example, confidentiality, equality, autonomy and others. Individuals should decide for themselves if they want to be tested, without coercion. What's more, there could be discriminations in employment and health insurance.

What is your view on presymptomatic testing for cancers? What are the ethical and social issues surrounding testing for BRCA1 and BRCA2? Give examples to support your viewpoints.

Part 4 Mini-lecture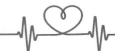

The Categories of Chunks (Idioms and Collocations)

Although English has the largest vocabulary among all languages in the world, there are many words in English we don't need at all. That is to say, there are many words that we need simply to understand when we read or hear them and seldom use them when we speak or write. On the other hand, there are words that we need to be able to use by ourselves, and the way we acquire these words certainly makes a difference. As advanced learners of English, we need to carefully study the way these words work with each other. There are different ways of categorizing chunks based on different conceptions and standards, and the chunks in this coursebook are divided into four categories, tailored to the needs of and convenience of learning for the college students. They are collocations, idioms and proverbs, sentence builders, and (sub)technical vocabulary.

Idioms (including proverbs which are whole clauses or sentences) are something that is of much interest to the learners, and we usually hope to use them skillfully in speeches and writings to show not only our linguistic but also cultural competence. Strictly speaking, idioms are a special type of collocations (which will be explained next). Understanding why idioms are "special" is important, as it gives hints to how to learn and use idioms properly.

First, most idioms are fixed in form. You are not allowed to change the words in an idiom. For example, you can only say somebody feels "on top of the world", but not "on top of the universe". By the same token, you describe somebody as "down-to-earth", but not "down-to-ground". Thus, when learning an idiom, you must carefully remember each and every word correctly. But sometimes you can vary the grammar in an idiom slightly. The active voice being changed into passive voice is a case in point. For example, "the director passed the buck to the sales manager" can be rewritten as "the buck was passed from the director to the sales manager".

Second, more often than not, the meaning of an idiom is not the sum of that of the individual words. The meaning of idioms describing happy feelings such as "walk on air" "on cloud nine" "over the moon" "in seventh heaven" is hardly evident from the words in them. Likewise, it's difficult to relate idioms such as "call a spade a spade" and "talk turkey" to the meaning of getting straight down to business. You should never underestimate the importance of acquiring cultural knowledge when learning an idiom since idioms are the carriers of cultural information. Besides, you should read more example sentences till you are certain of the precise meaning of an idiom. Many times, you need to try out with the native speakers and make progress by trials and errors.

Lastly, do not overburden your speaking and writing with idioms. A proper use of idioms and proverbs will definitely add color to your utterances and essays, and narrow the gap between you and your readers and listeners who are the native speakers of that language. But if you use too many in a speech or a short essay, it will backfire. So better use idioms in moderation and in the right settings.

The second category is collocations. A collocation is a natural combination of words. It suggests the way a word keeps another word or other words company. As mentioned earlier, it's a larger category which includes idioms in that a collocation is not that fixed in form. For example, words like "negative" "adverse", and "side" can all be combined with "effect" to mean the effect is undesirable. The word "change" can be followed by "seats" "schools" "jobs", and "places", all of which are viewed as natural and authentic English.

It's a worthwhile effort to have a good command of collocations because it usually distinguishes a good learner of English from a mediocre one. When you form a habit of keeping an eye on collocations, you are likely to speak and write more accurate and natural English. For example, when you say "make an order online", you may get the message across but it sounds odd and unidiomatic to a native ear, compared to "place an order online". So are "a high man" and "a tall mountain" compared to "a tall man" and "a high mountain". Besides, an excellent grasp of collocations can greatly enrich your vocabulary and avoid monotony and tediousness. We guess you may already have noticed that instead of saying that you are "happy" or "very happy", you can use a range of vocabulary and describe your happiness by saying that you are "on top of the world / on cloud nine / in seventh heaven".

We will discuss sentence builders and sub-technical chunks in Chapter 6.

Chapter 5

Alternative Medicine

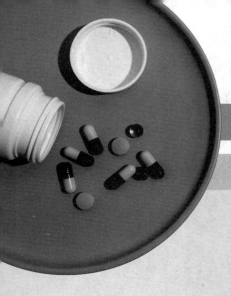

Chapter 5

Alternative Medicine

Learning Objectives

- to master some basic skills to build medical words with affixes concerning alternative medicine and to expand accurate usage of amphibious words in both general and medical contexts;

- to improve comprehensive linguistic abilities to discuss some methods used in alternative medicine;

- to compare and contrast modern medicine and alternative medicine, and to increase awareness of the benefits of the latter to man's general well-being.

Part 1 Pre-reading Tasks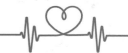

Task 1 Compare and Contrast

*Directions: In medical English, **amphibious words**, a term derived from amphibious animals such as frogs and toads that can live both on land and in water, have flexible meanings in both general contexts and medical contexts. Please consult your dictionaries, write down the Chinese equivalents of the amphibious words in the table below, and pay attention to their different meanings used as **general expressions (GE)** and **medical expressions (ME)** respectively. The first one is exemplified for you to follow.*

Amphibious Words	GE	ME
terminal	末端的，终点的	（疾病）晚期的
capsule		
concentration		
consolidate		
contract		

(Continued)

Amphibious Words	GE	ME
dysfunction		
develop		
infusion		
mixture		
tone		

Task 2 Read and Translate

Directions: Please read the following 10 pairs of sentences, and keep an eye on the 10 amphibious words you learned from the table in Task 1, which are interpreted differently as GE and ME. Translate the English sentences into Chinese.

1. The bus shuttles passengers back and forth from the station to the terminal. (GE)

   _____

   _____

   Some patients in the terminal stage of cancer recover miraculously. (ME)

   _____

   _____

2. The Dragon capsule is designed to be able to carry both astronauts and cargo. (GE)

   _____

   _____

   Aromatic capsules are great for easing the discomfort of a stuffy nose. (ME)

   _____

   _____

3. It requires considerable concentration to maintain a false breathing rate. (GE)

   _____

   _____

   In contrast, the drug with higher molecular weight tends to accumulate and maintain an effective concentration in tumor for a longer period. (ME)

_____

_____

4. She consolidated her power during her first year in office. (GE)

_____

_____

The sour taste of herbs has the property of constricting or consolidating. (ME)

_____

_____

5. We are in competition with four other companies for the contract. (GE)

_____

_____

A few individuals without this protein have contracted and even died from AIDS. (ME)

_____

_____

6. His severe emotional dysfunction was very apparent in the first semester as a freshman. (GE)

_____

_____

Thyroid dysfunction can also manifest in growing children in the form of mental and physical retardation. (ME)

_____

_____

7. Limited resources are restricting our capacity for developing new products. (GE)

_____

_____

He developed full-blown AIDS five years after contracting HIV. (ME)

_____

_____

8. But our traditional primary school English teaching makes the students learn by rote and infusion. (GE)

_____

_____

Intravenous infusions are also used to administer medications. (ME)

_____

_____

9. A mixture of skill and good luck decided the outcome of the game. (GE)

_____

_____

The Chinese herbal mixture has a variety of pharmacological effects in the treatment of viral pneumonia. (ME)

_____

_____

10. The article was moderate in tone and presented both sides of the case. (GE)

_____

_____

Massage will help to tone up loose skin under the chin. (ME)

_____

_____

Task 3 Lead-in Questions

Directions: Read the questions below and answer them in details.

1. Nowadays a lot of people prefer alternative medicine. What does the word "alternative" mean?

_____

_____

2. How many types of alternative medicine do you know? Please briefly describe each of them.

_____

_____

3. TCM (traditional Chinese medicine) has been gaining popularity worldwide over the past few decades thanks to its scientific nature and unique effectiveness. Do you have a story to tell based on your personal TCM experience, including your family and friends?

_____

_____

4. Medicines, after all, may cause adverse reactions or side effects. In general, what are the advantages of alternative medicine over Western medical systems?

_____

_____

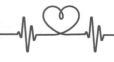

Part 2　Texts

Text A

Herbal Therapy

1　Together with ¹acupuncture, ²herbal medicine is a major ³pillar of **traditional Chinese medicine**. The Chinese ⁴pharmacopoeia lists over 6,000 different ⁵medicinal substances in terms of their properties and the ⁶disharmonies that they are helpful with. There are about 800 different herbs in common use today.

2　Herbs are classified in two major dimensions. The first dimension refers to the temperature characteristics of the herb, namely hot, warm, cold, neutral, and

[7]aromatic. The second refers to the taste properties of the herb, namely sour, bitter, sweet, spicy, and salty.

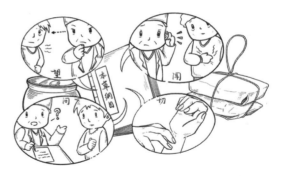

3   The various combinations of temperature and taste give the herbs properties that can influence the yin and yang energy patterns of the body. For example, sour, bitter and salty tastes are related to yin, whereas [8]acrid and sweet **are** [9]**attributed to** yang. There are herbs that will warm, or cool, or [10]tonify, or move stagnation and so on. Instead of possessing one quality, herbs are most always a combination of properties and temperatures and may reach one to as many as twelve organ systems. Warm herbs can be used with individuals suffering from heat disorders, but they must be mixed with herbs with cool or cold energy so that the overall balance of the mixture is on the cool side. Likewise, cool herbs can be used with people with cold disorders **as long as** the overall balance of the mixture is warm. Neutral herbs are neither hot nor cold, and are not too many in the pharmacopoeia.

4   As for the tastes, sour [11]constricts or [12]consolidates. Herbs of sour taste are often [13]indicated for use in [14]perspiration due to deficiency, [15]protracted cough, **chronic** [16]**diarrhea**, and other conditions related to [17]hypo-metabolism.

5   Bitter possesses the function of clearing heat, [18]purging the [19]bowels, lowering the [20]**qi**, improving appetite and drying dampness. Bitter herbs are commonly used in the acute stage of infectious diseases, and patterns of damp-heat or damp-cold, such as in [21]arthritis or [22]leucorrhoea.

6   Sweet has the function of [23]toning, improving, [24]moistening and [25]harmonizing many of the important systems of the body, including the digestive, respiratory, immune and [26]**endocrine systems**. Sweet tastes also relieve urgency and inhibit pain due to the constrictive action of muscles. They are commonly used for treating deficiency patterns such as dry cough, and [27]dysfunction of the **gastro-intestinal** [28]**tract** such as spleen and stomach disharmony.

7   Spicy [29]disperses, circulates qi and [30]vitalizes blood. This group of herbs can stimulate the **sweat** [31]**glands** to perspire, circulate qi, activate the function of organs and vitalize blood to promote **blood** [32]**circulation**. As a whole, spicy herbs have the overall effect of activating and enhancing metabolism. Spicy herbs are commonly used in the treatment of external patterns (catching a cold), when the function of the organs is weakened and circulation of blood has been [33]impeded. In traditional Chinese medical [34]terminology, this is the stage of **qi** [35]**stagnation and blood cloudiness**.

8   Salty herbs have the function of softening firm masses and [36]fibrous [37]adhesions. The salty taste purges and opens the bowels. Salty [38]agents are often indicated in sores, [39]inflammatory masses, [40]cysts, and **connective tissue** [41]**proliferation**.

9   The unique characteristic of Chinese herbal medicine is the degree to which [42]formulation is done. In Western herbal medicine, herbs are often delivered singly or combined into very small [43]formulas of herbs with the same function. **In contrast**, Chinese herbalists rarely prescribe a single herb to treat a condition. They create formulas instead. A formula usually contains at least four to twenty herbs.

10   **Herbal formulas** can be delivered **in all manner of** preparation. Pre-made formulas are available as pills, tablets, capsules, powders, water-[44]extracts, etc. Most of these formulas are very convenient as they do not [45]necessitate patient preparation and are easily taken. However, the [46]concentration of the herbs in these products is low and doesn't allow the practitioner to adjust the contents or [47]dosages. These products are usually not as [48]potent as the traditional preparation of [49]decoction.

11   Decoction is the traditional method of preparing herbal medicine. The practitioner weighs out a day's dosage of each herb and combines them in a bag. A patient is given a bag for each day the herbal formula will be taken. The herbs are then boiled in water by the patient at home. The boiling process takes 30 to 60 minutes and the resulting decoction will be consumed several times during the day.

12   Another modern way of delivering herbs is through [50]granulated herbs, which are highly concentrated powdered extracts. These powders are made by first preparing the herbs as a traditional decoction. The decoction is then dehydrated and the practitioners mix the powder [51]residue for each patient into a formula. The powder is then placed in hot water to recreate the decoction. This eliminates the need to prepare the herbs at home, but still retains much of the original decoction's potency.

Anon. 2003. Herbal therapy. Tcmpage. Retrieved and adapted on September 20, 2022, from Tcmpage website.

(796 words)

Notes

1. (Para. 1) acupuncture：针刺疗法。针灸由针法（acupuncture）和灸法（moxi-bustion）构成，是东方医学的重要组成部分之一。针法是指在中医理论的指导下把针具（通常指毫针）按照一定的角度刺入患者体内，运用捻转与提插等针刺手法来对人体特定部位进行刺激从而达到治疗疾病的目的。刺入点被称为人体腧穴，简称穴位。灸法是以预制的灸炷或灸草在体表一定的穴位上烧灼、熏熨，利用热的刺激来预防和治疗疾病；通常以艾草最为常用，故而称为艾灸，另有隔药灸、柳条灸、灯芯灸、桑枝灸等方法。

2. (Para. 1) The Chinese pharmacopoeia lists over 6,000 different medicinal substances in terms of their properties and the disharmonies that they are helpful with. 中国的药典按性状和治疗的症状列举了超过 6 000 种药物。
   pharmacopoeia：药典，是一个国家收录、记载药品规格、制备工艺、检验标准的法典。一般来说，一个国家的药典只收录那些药效确切、副作用小、品质稳定的药物及其制剂，并对其品质标准、制备要求、鉴别、杂质检查、含量测定作出具有法律效力的规定。

3. (Para. 3) The various combinations of temperature and taste give the herbs properties that can influence the yin and yang energy patterns of the body. 气与味的不同组合让草药具有影响身体阴阳能量模式的属性。
   temperature and taste：（中药的）气与味，是传统的中药分类依据。四气五味是中药药性理论的基本内容之一，最早载于《神农本草经》，其序录云：“药有酸咸甘苦辛五味，又有寒热温凉四气。”

4. (Para. 6) Sweet tastes also relieve urgency and inhibit pain due to the constrictive action of muscles. 甘味也能起缓和作用，或抑制肌肉收缩引起的疼痛。

5. (Para. 6) deficiency patterns：虚症，指人体阴阳、气血、津液、精髓等正气亏虚，而邪气不显著，表现为不足、松弛、衰退等征候。虚症主要分为阴虚、气虚、血虚和阳虚，其表现出来的症状有很大差异，要分清其类型，然后针对性进补。

6. (Para. 8) Salty agents are often indicated in sores, inflammatory masses, cysts, and connective tissue proliferation. 咸味药剂经常用于疮、炎症肿块、囊肿和结缔组织增生的治疗。
   1）agent：在此句语境中为“药剂”之意。
   2）cyst：囊肿。
   3）connective tissue proliferation：结缔组织增生。

7. (Para. 10) Most of these formulas are very convenient as they do not necessitate patient preparation and are easily taken. 这些药方大都方便使用，不需要病人花长时间制备，也易于服用。

1）necessitate：使……成为必需。

2）此句中，as 引导原因状语，解释"方便使用"的原因。

8. (Para. 12) The decoction is then dehydrated and the practitioners mix the powder residue for each patient into a formula. 煎制的药汤做脱水处理，药师把干燥的粉末按处方混合，发给病人。

dehydrate：使……脱水。

Word List

1. **acupuncture** ['ækjʊˌpʌŋktʃər] *n.*
   the treatment of a person's illness or pain by sticking small needles into their body at certain places 针灸，针刺疗法

2. **herbal** ['hɜːrb(ə)l] *adj.*
   connected with or made from herbs 药草的，香草的

3. **pillar** ['pɪlər] *n.*
   a basic part or feature of a system, organization, etc. 核心，支柱

4. **pharmacopoeia** [ˌfɑːməkə'piːə] *n.*
   an official book containing a list of medicines and drugs and instructions for their use 药典

5. **medicinal** [mə'dɪsən(ə)l] *adj.*
   helpful in the process of healing illness or infection 有疗效的，药用的

6. **disharmony** [dɪs'hɑːmənɪ] *n.*
   the lack of harmony 失调

7. **aromatic** [ˌærə'mætɪk] *adj.*
   having a pleasant noticeable smell 芳香的

8. **acrid** ['ækrɪd] *adj.*
   having a strong, bitter smell or taste that is usually unpleasant 辛辣的，刺激的

9. **attribute** [ə'trɪbjuːt] *v.*
   to explain by indicating a cause 把……归因于

10. **tonify** ['təʊnɪfaɪ] *v.*
    to make a part of the body firmer, smoother and stronger, by exercise or by applying special creams, etc. 改善（身体部位的）状况

11. **constrict** [kən'strɪkt] *v.*
    to make sth. tighter or narrower 紧缩

12. **consolidate** [kən'sɑːlɪdeɪt] *v.*

    to make sth. stronger 使……结实；巩固

13. **indicate** ['ɪndɪkeɪt] *v.*

    (usually passive) to be necessary or recommended 有必要，被建议

14. **perspiration** [ˌpɜːrspə'reɪʃ(ə)n] *n.*

    the action or process of perspiring 排汗，出汗

15. **protracted** [prə'træktɪd] *adj.*

    lasting longer than expected or longer than usual 延长的，持久的

16. **diarrhea** [daɪə'riːə] *n.*

    frequent and watery bowel movements 腹泻

17. **hypo-metabolism** [ˌhaɪpəme'tæbəlɪzəm] *n.*

    the condition in which metabolism is less effective than usual 新陈代谢减退，新陈代谢不足

18. **purge** [pɜːrdʒ] *v.*

    to evacuate one's bowels 催泄，通便

19. **bowel** ['baʊəl] *n.*

    the tube along which food passes after it has been through the stomach 肠

20. **qi** [tʃiː] *n.*

    (in Oriental medicine, martial arts, etc.) vital energy believed to circulate round the body in currents 气

21. **arthritis** [ɑːr'θraɪtɪs] *n.*

    a disease that causes pain and swelling in one or more joints of the body 关节炎

22. **leucorrhoea** [ljuːkə'riːə] *n.*

    a white or yellowish discharge of mucous material from the vagina, often an indication of infection 白带

23. **tone** [təʊn] *v.*

    to make your muscles, skin, etc. firmer and stronger 使……更健壮，使……更有力

24. **moisten** ['mɔɪs(ə)n] *v.*

    to make sth. slightly wet 使……湿润

25. **harmonize** ['hɑːrmənaɪz] *v.*

    to make sth. in harmony 使……协调，使……和谐

26. **endocrine** ['endəkrɪn] *adj.*

    of or relating to glands that put hormones and other products directly into the blood 内分泌的

27. **dysfunction** [dɪs'fʌŋkʃ(ə)n] *n.*

any disturbance in the functioning of an organ or body part 功能紊乱，机能障碍

28. **tract** [trækt] *n.*

a system of connected organs or tissues along which materials or messages pass 道

29. **disperse** [dɪ'spɜːrs] *v.*

to make sth. spread over a wide area 使……分散

30. **vitalize** ['vaɪtəˌlaɪz] *v.*

to make vital, living, or alive; to endow with life or vigor 使……有生气，给……活力

31. **gland** [glænd] *n.*

an organ in a person's or an animal's body that produces a substance for the body to use 腺

32. **circulation** [ˌsɜːrkjə'leɪʃ(ə)n] *n.*

the movement of blood around the body 血液循环

33. **impede** [ɪm'piːd] *v.*

to delay or stop the progress of sth. 阻碍，阻止

34. **terminology** [ˌtɜːrmɪ'nɑːlədʒɪ] *n.*

the set of technical words or expressions used in a particular subject 术语

35. **stagnation** [stæg'neɪʃ(ə)n] *n.*

inactivity 停滞，不流动

36. **fibrous** ['faɪbrəs] *adj.*

made of many fibers; looking like fibers 由纤维构成的，纤维状的

37. **adhesion** [æd'hiːʒ(ə)n] *n.*

a piece of tissue that grows around a cut or diseased area 粘连

38. **agent** ['eɪdʒənt] *n.*

a chemical or a substance that produces an effect or is used for a particular purpose 药剂

39. **inflammatory** [ɪn'flæmətɔːrɪ] *adj.*

causing or involving inflammation 发炎的，炎性的

40. **cyst** [sɪst] *n.*

a growth containing liquid that forms in or on a person's or an animal's body and may need to be removed 囊肿

41. proliferation [prəˌlɪfə'reɪʃ(ə)n] *n.*

rapid reproduction of a cell, part, or organism 增生

42. formulation [ˌfɔːmjʊ'leɪʃ(ə)n] *n.*

the way in which different ingredients are combined to make a medicine 配方

43. formula ['fɔːrmjələ] *n.*

(*pl.* formulas/formulae) a list of the things that sth. is made from, giving the amount of each substance to use 配方，处方

44. extract ['ekstrækt] *n.*

a substance that has been obtained from sth. else using a particular process 提取物，浓缩物

45. necessitate [nə'sesɪteɪt] *v.*

to make sth. necessary 使……成为必要

46. concentration [ˌkɑːns(ə)n'treɪʃ(ə)n] *n.*

the amount of a substance in a liquid or in another substance 浓度，含量

47. dosage ['dəʊsɪdʒ] *n.*

an amount of sth., usually a medicine or a drug, that is taken regularly over a particular period of time 剂量

48. potent ['pəʊtənt] *adj.*

having a strong effect on your body or mind 有强效的

49. decoction [dɪ'kɑːkʃ(ə)n] *n.*

the extraction of the water-soluble substances of a drug or medicinal plants by boiling 煎煮；汤剂，药汁

50. granulated ['grænjʊleɪtɪd] *adj.*

in the form of small grains 颗粒状的

51. residue ['rezɪduː] *n.*

a small amount of sth. that remains at the end of a process 残留物，残渣

Chunk List

Collocations

1. attribute... to... 把……归因于……

She attributes her success to hard work and a little luck.

她认为她的成功来自勤劳和一点好运气。

2. **in contrast** 与此相反，相比之下

In contrast, the lives of girls in rich families were often very sheltered.

相比之下，富裕家庭的女孩子们通常都过着养尊处优的生活。

Idioms and Proverbs

3. **as long as** 只要

We'll go, as long as the weather is good.

只要天气好，我们就去。

4. **in all manner of** 各种各样的，形形色色的

The problem can be solved in all manner of ways.

这个问题可以用各种方法加以解决。

(Sub)Technical Chunks

5. **traditional Chinese medicine (TCM)** 中医

The hospital of traditional Chinese medicine installed a computer to fill prescriptions.

这家中医医院装上了电子计算机来抓药。

6. **chronic diarrhea** 慢性腹泻

Symptoms of infection include chronic diarrhea and vomiting.

感染症状包括慢性腹泻和呕吐。

7. **endocrine system** 内分泌系统

The endocrine system is a system that acts on various organs throughout the body.

内分泌系统是一种作用于周身各器官的系统。

8. **gastro-intestinal tract** 胃肠道

This will allow the robot to crawl around the gastro-intestinal tract and perform treatment with appropriate surgical tools.

这将使机器人可以在胃肠道周围爬行，并用适当的外科手术工具施行治疗。

9. **sweat gland** 汗腺

The body relies on sweat glands to secrete a clear, potentially odorous substance onto the surface of the skin in order to reduce the body temperature.

身体依靠汗腺将一种透明的、可能有气味的物质分泌到皮肤表面来降低体温。

10. **blood circulation** 血液循环

Regular exercise will improve blood circulation.

经常锻炼会促进血液循环。

11. **qi stagnation and blood cloudiness** 气滞血浊

Qi stagnation and blood cloudiness are popular among young patients.

气滞血浊多见于青年患者。

12. **connective tissue proliferation** 结缔组织增生

The chronic rejection included connective tissue proliferation.

慢性排异反应包括结缔组织增生。

13. **herbal formula** 草药方剂，草本配方

Many Chinese trust in the curative effects of herbal formulas.

许多中国人信赖草药方剂的疗效。

Text B

Benefits of [1]Oncology [2]Massage

1   Many cancer centers now offer oncology massage as a [3]complementary treatment for cancer. In this sense, massage is not used as a treatment for cancer, but as a method of helping with the symptoms of cancer and the side effects of treatment.

2   The research is young, but oncology massage may help with pain control, mood disorders, cancer-related [4]fatigue, and **quality of life**. Massage may also play a role in the prevention of [5]**neuropathic pain** related to some chemotherapy drugs. Here we discuss each of them.

Pain Control

3   As with [6]nausea and vomiting, oncology massage should not be used to replace conventional treatments for pain, but help to reduce pain or the amount of **pain medication** people take. It may be especially helpful with pain due to surgery. The [7]mechanism isn't well understood, but massage has been found to increase the release of [8]endorphins, and increased levels of endorphins result in a reduction in pain. For example, neuropathic pain is common in people treated with the chemotherapy drug Taxol, and a 2019 study found that people who underwent classical

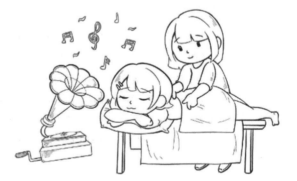

massage **prior to** a Taxol [9]infusion reported less pain. This was also seen objectively in nerve [10]conduction studies.

Mood Disorders

4   Several studies have found that oncology massage can reduce anxiety and **stresses and strains** for people living with cancer. In many cases, massage appears to lower [11]cortisol levels and the reduction of the **stress** [12]**hormones** possibly has other physical benefits as well. Decreased anxiety has been noted in a number of different studies.

5   Of all of the symptoms that massage may help with, depression and mood disorders have the **strongest evidence**. Depression and mood disorders are not only common in women with **breast cancer**, but are challenging for the doctors as many [13]antidepressants reduce the effectiveness of some breast cancer medications (such as Tamoxifen). In addition, a few studies have found that depression **is associated with** lower **survival rates** in women with breast cancer.

Cancer-related Fatigue

6   Massage has been found to reduce cancer fatigue in some people. While not a [14]life-threatening symptom, fatigue is one of the more annoying and frustrating symptoms for people with cancer and often [15]persists for years after treatment has been completed in those with early-stage disease.

Quality of Life

7   Unlike the often intense (and sometimes cold) nature of treatments such as chemotherapy and radiation, massage can lead to a sense of **peace and quiet**. In many cases, it may significantly reduce physical symptoms and improve quality of life. In addition, since much of cancer treatment is aimed at treating a tumor, massage can help people feel [16]pampered as the therapy involves a therapist **being devoted to** your personal and non-clinical [17]well-being.

8   Some studies evaluating the potential benefits of oncology massage have focused on specific treatments. For example, a 2016 study looked at the benefits of massage in people going through chemotherapy, finding that it led to relief of pain, fatigue, nausea, and anxiety. Besides, in the [18]**palliative care** setting, massage therapy may also be helpful. A 2019 study found that massage therapy enhanced well-being primarily by allowing people to have a break in which they could "escape" from their disease.

9   You may take some tips to make oncology massage more productive. **First and [19]foremost**, talk to your oncologist about any precautions or concerns he/she has. It's important to discuss any of this with your massage therapist, as well as any concerns you have about [20]lotions, oils, or [21]aromatherapy. Some therapists use aromatherapy with massage, and play [22]soothing music.

10   Next, you may be asked to remove your clothing except for your underwear, but this can vary. You should never feel uncomfortable, and a massage can be performed through clothing if you wish. You will usually be asked to lie on a cushioned table, with a special hole for your face when you lie on your stomach. Positioning may be limited or need to be altered. For example, if you've had recent breast cancer surgery, you may not be able to lie on your abdomen or one side.

11   Thirdly, when you are receiving a massage, make sure to let the therapist know if anything is painful, or if you need a more gentle touch. Being uncomfortable or experiencing pain is unnecessary for the massage to be effective and could be harmful instead. Most sessions last 30 minutes to 90 minutes, but you can ask the therapist to stop at any time.

12   **Last but not least**, when you get up after your massage, be careful standing. Some people become very relaxed and feel [23]light-headed when standing. Give yourself time to get up and get dressed.

Eldridge, L. 2022. Benefits and techniques of oncology massage—learn how massage therapy for people with cancer works. Verywellhealth. Retrieved and adapted on September 20, 2022, from Verywellhealth website.

(769 words)

Notes

1. (Para. 3) endorphin：内啡肽，亦称安多芬或脑内啡，是一种内成性（脑下垂体分泌）的类吗啡生物化学合成物激素。它是由脑下垂体和脊椎动物的丘脑下部所分泌的氨基化合物（肽）。它能与吗啡受体结合，产生跟吗啡、鸦片剂一样的止痛效果和欣快感，效果等同于天然的镇痛剂。利用药物可增加脑内啡肽的分泌效果。

2. (Para. 3) For example, neuropathic pain is common in people treated with the chemotherapy drug Taxol, and a 2019 study found that people who underwent classical massage prior to a Taxol infusion reported less pain. 比如，接受紫杉醇化疗的人常有神经性疼痛，而 2019 年的一项研究表明，在接受紫杉醇注射前接受古典式按摩的人的疼痛有所减轻。

Taxol：紫杉醇，是一种从裸子植物红豆杉的树皮分离提纯的天然次生代谢产物，也是天然的抗癌药物，分子式为 $C_{47}H_{51}NO_{14}$，在临床上已经广泛用于乳腺癌、卵巢癌和部分头颈癌和肺癌的治疗。

3. (Para. 4) In many cases, massage appears to lower cortisol levels and the reduction of the stress hormones possibly has other physical benefits as well. 在多数情况下，按摩可以降低皮质醇水平，而压力激素的减少可能对身体还有其他益处。

cortisol：皮质醇，是肾上腺皮质产生的一种激素，也叫压力激素。在压力状态下身体需要皮质醇来维持正常的生理机能。皮质醇升高时，患者可能会出现血压异常、满月脸、库欣综合征等；皮质醇降低时，患者可能会出现激素水平、血压水平、体温水平降低等。

4. (Para. 5) depression：抑郁症，是一种常见的精神障碍。当抑郁症反复发作，并达到中度或重度时，可能成为一种严重的健康疾患。在抑郁发作期间，患者连续两周以上几乎每天大部分时间都心情郁闷（感觉悲伤、烦躁、空虚），对活动丧失愉悦感或兴趣；还会出现其他一些症状，可能包括注意力不集中、过度内疚或自我贬低、对未来绝望、有死亡或自杀想法、睡眠紊乱、食欲或体重变化，以及感到特别劳累或缺乏精力。根据抑郁症发作的严重程度和类型，医生可以为患者提供心理治疗，如行为激活、认知行为疗法（CBT）和人际心理疗法（IPT），或者提供抗抑郁药，如选择性血清素再摄取抑制剂（SSRIs 类）和三环类抗抑郁药（TCAs 类）。

5. (Para. 6) While not a life-threatening symptom, fatigue is one of the more annoying and frustrating symptoms for people with cancer and often persists for years after treatment has been completed in those with early-stage disease. 疲惫乏力并非事关生死的症状，但却令癌症患者更为苦恼和沮丧，该症状通常会在早期癌症病人的治疗结束后仍持续数年。

6. (Para. 7) chemotherapy and radiation：化疗与放疗。化疗指化学疗法，采用向病人体内注射化疗药物的方法来杀死肿瘤，属于全身性的抗肿瘤治疗手段。放疗指放射治疗，用高能放射线杀死肿瘤，采用大型医疗设备加速器来完成，属于局部的抗肿瘤治疗办法。二者都属于治疗恶性肿瘤的常用手段，优点是可杀灭癌细胞、抑制其生长和繁殖，副作用是免疫功能下降、骨髓抑制等。

7. (Para. 7) In addition, since much of cancer treatment is aimed at treating a tumor, massage can help people feel pampered as the therapy involves a therapist being devoted to your personal and non-clinical well-being. 除此之外，由于多数癌症治疗都是治疗肿瘤，所以按摩可以使人们感受到关心、照顾，因为肿瘤按摩疗法的治疗师会致力于改善你个人的、非临床方面的健康状况。

8. (Para. 8) palliative care：安宁疗护，又称姑息治疗，是指为疾病终末期或老年患者在临终前提供身体、心理、精神等方面的照料和人文关怀等服务。此疗法通过控制痛苦和不适症状，提高生命质量，帮助患者舒适、安详、有尊严地离世。

9. (Para. 8) A 2019 study found that massage therapy enhanced well-being primarily by allowing people to have a break in which they could "escape" from their disease. 2019 年的一项研究发现，按摩疗法是通过让人们用短暂的休息时间暂时"逃离"疾病来改善他们身心状况的。

10. (Para. 10) You will usually be asked to lie on a cushioned table, with a special hole for your face when you lie on your stomach. 通常，治疗师会让你躺在有垫子的台子上，垫子上专门设有供俯卧时摆放脸部的孔洞。

    lie on one's stomach：俯卧。

Word List

1. **oncology** [ɑːnˈkɑːlədʒɪ] *n.*
    the scientific study of and treatment of tumors in the body 肿瘤学

2. **massage** [məˈsɑːʒ] *n.*
    the action of rubbing and pressing a person's body with the hands to reduce pain in the muscles and joints 按摩

3. **complementary** [ˌkɑːmplɪˈment(ə)rɪ] *adj.*
    treating patients in ways which are different from the ones used by most Western doctors, for example acupuncture 辅助性的

4. **fatigue** [fəˈtiːg] *n.*
    a feeling of being extremely tired, usually because of hard work or exercise 疲劳

5. **neuropathic** [ˌnjʊrəˈpæθɪk] *adj.*
    related to nerves 神经性的

6. **nausea** [ˈnɔːzɪə] *n.*
    the feeling that you have when you want to vomit, for example because you are ill/sick or are disgusted by sth. 恶心，作呕

7. **mechanism** [ˈmekənɪz(ə)m] *n.*
    a method or a system for achieving sth. 方法，机制

8. **endorphin** [enˈdɔːrfɪn] *n.*
    a hormone produced in the brain that reduces the feeling of pain 内啡肽

9. **infusion** [ɪnˈfjuːʒ(ə)n] *n.*
    an act of slowly putting a drug or other substance into a person's vein（药物等的）输注

10. **conduction** [kən'dʌkʃ(ə)n] *n.*

    the transmission 传导

11. **cortisol** ['kɔːrtɪsɒl] *n.*

    a hormone produced by the adrenal cortex, that regulates carbohydrate metabolism, maintains blood pressure and is released in response to stress 皮质醇

12. **hormone** ['hɔːrməʊn] *n.*

    a chemical substance produced in the body or in a plant that encourages growth or influences how the cells and tissues function 激素

13. **antidepressant** [ˌæntɪdɪ'pres(ə)nt] *n.*

    a drug used to treat depression 抗抑郁药

14. **life-threatening** ['laɪf ˌθretnɪŋ] *adj.*

    that is likely to kill sb. 可能致命的，危及生命的

15. **persist** [pər'sɪst] *v.*

    to continue to exist 保持，持续存在

16. **pampered** ['pæmpərd] *adj.*

    being treated with extreme or excessive care and attention 被溺爱的，被细心照顾的

17. **well-being** [ˌwel 'biːɪŋ] *n.*

    general health and happiness 健康，安乐

18. **palliative** ['pælɪətɪv] *adj.*

    relieving pain or alleviating a problem without dealing with the underlying cause 减轻痛苦的，缓解的

19. **foremost** ['fɔːrməʊst] *adv.*

    most importantly 最重要地

20. **lotion** ['ləʊʃ(ə)n] *n.*

    a liquid used for cleaning, protecting or treating the skin 洁肤液，护肤液

21. **aromatherapy** [əˌrəʊmə'θerəpɪ] *n.*

    the use of natural oils that smell sweet for controlling pain or for rubbing into the body during massage 芳香疗法

22. **soothing** ['suːðɪŋ] *adj.*

    making sb. who is anxious, upset, etc. feel calmer 舒缓的

23. **light-headed** [ˌlaɪt 'hedɪd] *adj.*

    not completely in control of your thoughts or movements; slightly fain 头晕的，眩晕的

Chunk List

Collocations

1. **quality of life** 生活质量
    His quality of life has improved dramatically since the operation.
    手术后，他的生活质量大大改善了。

2. **prior to** 在……前
    A death prior to 65 is considered to be a premature death.
    65 岁以前死亡被认为是过早死亡。

3. **stresses and strains** 压力
    You will learn to cope with the stresses and strains of the job.
    你将学会怎样应对这项工作的紧张与压力。

4. **strong evidence** 有力证据
    There is strong evidence of a link between exercise and a healthy heart.
    有充分的证据证明锻炼与心脏健康有关系。

5. **be associated with** 与……相联系
    These symptoms are particularly associated with depression.
    这些症状尤其与抑郁症相关联。

6. **survival rate** 存活率
    Maternal age affects the baby's survival rate.
    母亲（生育时）的年龄影响婴儿的成活率。

7. **peace and quiet** 安静，宁静
    I would work better if I had some peace and quiet.
    四周要是再安静一些，我会干得更好。

8. **be devoted to** 专心于，致力于
    My father has been devoted to the cause of education for many years.
    我父亲多年来一直致力于教育事业。

Idioms and Proverbs

9. **first and foremost** 首要的是，首先
    He does a little teaching, but first and foremost he's a writer.
    他承担一点教学工作，但首要的身份是作家。

10. **last but not least** 最后但同样重要的是
    Last but not least, I'd like to thank all the catering staff.
    最后但同样重要的是，我要感谢所有的餐饮工作人员。

(Sub)Technical Chunks

11. **neuropathic pain** 神经性疼痛

    Neuropathic pain is driven by nerves gone wrong.

    神经性疼痛是由神经紊乱造成的。

12. **pain medication** 止痛药

    This not only helps relieve anxiety, but reduces the need for pain medication as well.

    这不仅能够降低焦虑，还能减少病人对止痛药的需求。

13. **stress hormone** 压力激素

    Laughing lowers levels of stress hormones and strengthens the immune system.

    笑可以降低压力激素水平并增强免疫系统。

14. **breast cancer** 乳腺癌

    Breast cancer is the most common form of cancer among women in this country.

    乳腺癌是这个国家妇女中最常见的一种癌症。

15. **palliative care** 姑息治疗，保守治疗

    In line with almost every other form of medical care, palliative care has its limits.

    同几乎任何其他疗法一样，姑息疗法也有自身的局限性。

Part 3 Post-reading Exercises

3.1 Read and Answer

3.1.1 Directions: Read Text A in Part 2 and choose the best answers to the following questions.

1. Which of the following does NOT belong to traditional Chinese medicine?

    A. Massage.

    B. Acupuncture.

    C. Herbal medicine.

    D. Laser therapy.

2. How can herbs be classified according to the text?

    A. By temperature or taste.

    B. By shape.

    C. By color.

    D. By weight.

3. Which of the following is true according to the text?
    A. The yin and yang energy patterns of the body can not be changed.
    B. Sour, salty and sweet tastes are related to yin.
    C. People with heat disorders may use warm herbs.
    D. Bitter and acrid are related to yang.

4. From Paragraph 3 we can infer that _____.
    A. warm herbs can not be mixed with cold herbs
    B. herbs can be mixed to reach the overall balance to cure some diseases
    C. neutral herbs are either hot or cold
    D. cool herbs can be used for people with heat disorders

5. Which of the following taste-disease matches is FALSE according to the text?
    A. Sour—diarrhea.
    B. Bitter—arthritis.
    C. Sweet—dysfunction of spleen.
    D. Spicy—cough.

6. What's special about Chinese herbal medicine?
    A. Formulas are used to treat diseases.
    B. Herbs are often delivered singly.
    C. A formula usually contains four to twelve herbs.
    D. Herbs with the same function are combined into small formulas.

7. The following are all available forms of pre-made formulas EXCEPT _____.
    A. powders
    B. capsules
    C. gases
    D. water-extracts

8. Which of the following is NOT a disadvantage of pre-made herbal formulas?
    A. The concentration of the herbs in products such as pills and tablets is low.
    B. Contents or dosages can not be adjusted.
    C. They can be taken with great ease.
    D. The products are not as effective as traditionally prepared decoctions.

9. What's the advantage of preparing herbal medicine through granulated herbs over decoction?
    A. The boiling process takes less than 30 minutes.
    B. Patients don't need to boil the herbs at home.
    C. It does not need the process of decoction.
    D. It loses much of the original decoction's potency.

10. What is the main idea of the text?

    A. An introduction to traditional Chinese medicine.

    B. A comparison between Chinese and Western herbal medicine.

    C. The functions of different tastes of herbs.

    D. An introduction to herbal medicine from different aspects.

3.1.2 **Directions:** *Read Text B in Part 2 and finish the following exercises. Write T for True, F for False, or NG for Not Given in the brackets before the statements based on the instructions below.*

True	*if the statement agrees with the claims of the author;*
False	*if the statement contradicts the claims of the author;*
Not Given	*if it is impossible to say what the author thinks about it.*

(   ) 1. Oncology massage can be used to cure cancer.

(   ) 2. Though the research of oncology massage is young, it proves to have many advantages.

(   ) 3. Conventional treatments for pain can sometimes be replaced by oncology massage.

(   ) 4. Massage can best help with depression and mood disorders.

(   ) 5. Fatigue can disappear instantly after treatment in patients with early-stage cancer.

(   ) 6. Massage can be useful and effective both physically and mentally.

(   ) 7. The skills of the massage therapist have an influence on people's experience.

(   ) 8. You must keep silent when receiving a massage.

(   ) 9. You can ask the massage therapist to stop at any time.

(   ) 10. If you've had recent liver cancer, you can't receive a massage.

3.2 Guess and Choose

Directions: *Figure out the meanings of the following medical affixes and choose the best answer from the four choices marked A, B, C and D.*

1. hypo (   )

    A. high   B. super   C. heavy   D. beneath or low

2. hydr, hydro (   )

    A. hygiene   B. hybrid   C. water or hydrogen   D. hysteria

3. fibr, fibro (   )
   A. fiber   B. fight   C. fix   D. fist

4. dys (   )
   A. dislike   B. difficult   C. different   D. delight

5. granul, granulo (   )
   A. powder   B. gravity   C. particle   D. gradual

6. logy (   )
   A. logic   B. log   C. logo   D. a branch of science

7. meta (   )
   A. after or beyond B. metaphor   C. metal   D. mental

8. endo (   )
   A. endow   B. endorse   C. internal   D. external

9. colon, colono (   )
   A. a mark following a list   B. large intestine
   C. small intestine   D. abdomen

10. ia, iasis, osis (   )
    A. medical condition   B. air sacs
    C. digestion   D. airway

3.3 **Read and Think**

Directions: Read the following medical words built with the medical affixes from Exercise 3.2 and write down their Chinese equivalents in the table below.

Terminology	Chinese Equivalents	Terminology	Chinese Equivalents
hypo-metabolism		**hypo**tension	
de**hydr**ate		**hydro**gen	
fibrous		**fiber**	
dysfunction		**dys**pnea	
granulated		**granul**oma	
termino**logy**		geronto**logy**	
metabolic		**meta**bolism	
endorphin		**endo**crine	
colon		**colono**scopy	
dyspeps**ia**		thromb**osis**	

3.4 Match and Fill

3.4.1 Directions: *Match the medical terms (a–j) in the box below with their definitions (1–10).*

a. acupuncture	b. disharmony	c. tonify	d. dysfunction
e. practitioner	f. oncology	g. neuropathic	h. chemotherapy
i. antidepressant	j. palliative		

(   ) 1. abnormal or impaired functioning of a bodily system or organ

(   ) 2. the branch of medicine that deals with tumors, including study of their development, diagnosis, treatment, and prevention

(   ) 3. the use of sharp, thin needles that are inserted in the body at very specific points

(   ) 4. treatment of cancer with anticancer drugs

(   ) 5. the loss of balance

(   ) 6. to make a part of the body firmer, smoother, and stronger, by exercise or by applying special creams, etc.

(   ) 7. a drug used to treat depression

(   ) 8. relating to any disease of the nerves

(   ) 9. a person who practices medicine

(   ) 10. a medicine or medical treatment that reduces pain without curing its cause

3.4.2 Directions: *Make good use of the medical terms you learned from Exercise 3.4.1 and fill in the blanks in the sentences below. Change the form where necessary.*

1. Without sleep, our body's clock loses its rhythm and starts to _____, causing poor habits.

2. To _____ qi of the kidney is good for health.

3. Breast cancer is one of the most common harmful tumors, and it is the hotspot and focus of _____ field at all times.

4. Traditional Chinese doctors have practiced _____ for centuries.

5. Depression may play a role in weight gain due to adverse effects of _____ drugs.

6. _____ pain is a familiar sight of many patients and it can be suffering.

7. I was visiting a dear young friend in the _____ care unit in our local hospital.

8. For those who are ill, illness is an internal form of _____.

9. He lost all his hair due to the side effects of the _____.

10. You're likely to start by first seeing your family doctor or a general _____.

3.5 Fill and Translate

3.5.1 *Directions: Choose the correct medical words from the box below to fill in the gaps (1–10) of the passage concerning traditional Chinese medicine. Change the form where necessary.*

acupuncture	agent	asthma	heal	harmony
herb	massage	pharmacopoeia	practitioner	prescribe

China has one of the world's oldest medical systems. Traditional Chinese medicine is a system of medicine which is at least 23 centuries old. The TCM practitioners seek to restore a dynamic balance between two complementary forces, yin (passive) and yang (active), which pervade the human body as they do the universe as a whole. According to TCM, a person is healthy when (1) _____ exists between these two forces; illness, on the other hand, results from a breakdown in the balance of yin and yang. A visit to a traditional Chinese pharmacy is like a visit to a small natural history museum. The hundreds of cabinet drawers, glass cases, and jars in a typical pharmacy hold an enormous variety of desiccated plant and animal material. To restore harmony, the practitioner may use any of a large array of traditional remedies. The patient may be treated with acupuncture, moxa treatment, or cupping (using hot glass cups to draw blood to the skin).

A TCM practitioner uses smell, hearing, touch, and pulse diagnosis to discover the source of an unbalanced health condition. Usually, the patient will get a(n) (2) _____ formula prepared with one of thousands of plants or dried animal parts in the Chinese (3) _____. An understanding of the essence of various (4) _____ components gives the TCM practitioner a way to create a healing effect that reaches beyond the chemical composition and physical properties of the herbs. The (5) _____ chooses the herbal formula whose essence correctly stimulates or adjusts the body's own energy vibration.

The TCM practitioner may also use (6) _____, in which thin needles are inserted into specific points along the meridians to alleviate symptoms. The needles stimulate the meridians to balance the body's yin and yang. In place of needles, (7) _____ can also be used to stimulate the acupuncture points. Acupuncture is sometimes accompanied by moxa treatment, the burning of small cones of an herb

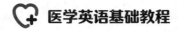

at acupuncture points.

Various Western scientific disciplines have conducted studies to learn how Chinese medicine works. Nearly 200 modern medicines have been developed either directly or indirectly from the 7,300 species of plants used as medicines in China. For example, ephedrine, an alkaloid used in treating (8) _____, was first isolated from the Chinese herb mahuang. Today, scientists continue to identify compounds in Chinese herbal remedies that may be useful in the development of some new therapeutic (9) _____.

However, sometimes it is difficult to use a Western way to measure Eastern medicine. For example, many studies on acupuncture involve research that attempts to prove that this modality can eliminate or reduce pain or alleviate certain conditions. However, this elementary approach ignores the deeper insight and experience of Chinese medicine that the human body has unlimited (10) _____ power and that the complementary energies of health and disease reflect the yinyang principle within the human body.

3.5.2 Directions: *Translate the underlined sentences from the passage above.*

1. A visit to a traditional Chinese pharmacy is like a visit to a small natural history museum.

   _____

   _____

2. To restore harmony, the practitioner may use any of a large array of traditional remedies.

   _____

   _____

3. A TCM practitioner uses smell, hearing, touch, and pulse diagnosis to discover the source of an unbalanced health condition.

   _____

   _____

4. Acupuncture is sometimes accompanied by moxa treatment, the burning of small cones of an herb at acupuncture points.

   _____

   _____

5. Nearly 200 modern medicines have been developed either directly or indirectly from the 7,300 species of plants used as medicines in China.

_____

_____

3.6 Speak and Write

3.6.1 Directions: *Discuss with your group members the phenomenon described in Topic 1 below, and select a representative to report your main ideas to the class.*

Topic 1

Many people think that using plants to treat illnesses is safer than taking medicine. People have been using plants in folk medicine for centuries. Yet "natural" does not mean safe. Some herbs can interact with other medicines or be toxic at high doses. In Western herbal medicine, herbs are often delivered singly or combined into very small formulas of herbs with the same function. In contrast, Chinese herbalists create formulas instead which usually contain at least four to twenty herbs. What Chinese philosophy can you tell that lies behind Chinese herbal formulas and the manners of preparation?

3.6.2 Directions: *Discuss with your group members the phenomenon described in Topic 2 below, and write an essay in about 160 words, entitled "The Cultural Differences as Reflected in Different Attitudes to Guasha".*

Topic 2

Guasha, or scraping massage, has been used as an ancient healing technique in China for centuries. It involves a massage tool to exert short or long strokes on the skin which stimulate the soft tissue on the skin to improve blood flow and circulation. However, the possible results from the scraping massage like bruising, pain, skin rashes, burst capillaries and bleeding scare the Westerners away. In their eyes, instead of wiping away aches, guasha shifts the pain, and only gives the patient mental comforts. The conflict is vividly revealed in the film *Guasha* directed by Zheng Xiaolong, in which this scraping massage is taken as domestic violence and child abuse in America.

Discuss the phenomenon with your group members, and analyze the Chinese wisdom reflected in guasha and the cautions we should exercise while applying the scraping massage on patients. Give examples to support your viewpoints.

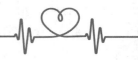

Part 4 Mini-lecture

Binomials

What is a binomial? It is an expression where two words are joined by a conjunctive (usually "and"), and the order of the two words are often fixed and can not be reversed at will. Roughly, we could say the pattern of a binomial is "word A + word B".

There are some clues that will help you to identify a binomial. An obvious criterion is the sound patterns, such as alliteration (the use of the same letter or sound at the beginning of the words) and rhyme (the use of the same sound at the end of the words). Please read the following examples and feel the power rendered by the sound effect when getting the message across.

Alliteration:

- They maintain the closest relations with the masses and share their **weal and woe**.
- Keeping the accounts is **part and parcel** of her job.
- The poor child was beaten **black and blue** by his drunk uncle.
- Life is no bed of roses; it's full of **trials and tribulations.**

Rhyme:

- We have nothing to worry about; it's a **fair and square** competition from start to finish.
- She's known as a prophet of **doom and groom.**
- Working in the PR (Public Relations) department, she always has to **wine and dine** her clients.
- Sometimes the **hustle and bustle** of the city just gets me down, so I escape to the countryside to enjoy some peace and quiet.

Synonymy (using words with the same or similar meanings) is another important clue.

- Students need to learn important skills such as teamwork and respect for **law and order.**
- We're relieved to hear that you are **safe and sound** after such an arduous journey.

- One of the recipes to a successful job interview is that you dress properly and look **clean and tidy.**
- Our neurological understanding of memory has advanced by **leaps and bounds** over the past decades.

Other times, you will find that word A and word B are grammar words instead of notional words.

- He is generally self-disciplined and works hard, but he needs a nudge **now and then.**
- It rained **on and off** last week.
- Bob was laid off due to the economic recession and currently becomes **down and out.**
- It's a beautiful boulevard and lined with cafes **here and there.**

Please remember that in a binomial, the conjunctive is not always the word "and". Besides, word A and word B can sometimes be antonyms (words having opposite meanings) instead of synonyms.

- To a retail business, location is always the golden rule. It determines whether that business will **sink or swim.**
- There is no clear **right or wrong** solution to this tricky problem.
- In previous trade rounds, the large corporations set the rules and the small ones could only **take it or leave it.**
- They sat for hours debating the **pros and cons** of setting up their own firm.

Now that you have had some idea about binomials, you may have already grown an interest in this special language phenomenon. You may even be impressed by the beauty and power of binomials and want to use them on your own. Here're some suggestions for you to take. First, try to increase your consciousness (or stay alert) when you come across binomials in your reading and listening in the future. Second, try to have some feel about how it pays dividends in your communication when you speak and write binomials. It is generally accepted that proper use of binomials in speaking and writing will not only add a color to the message you want to convey, but also make the message more memorable, and your communication more efficient and effective. Therefore, third, why not form a habit of copying down the binomials in your notebooks from now on? You need to build your reservoir and it will be proven a worthwhile effort. Last but not least, we suggest you organize your binomials in line with the clues (or criteria) we have listed above. There's a real plus when you arrange your copied-down binomials in an apple-pie form, as this will render it easy to remember and quick to retrieve them in real use.

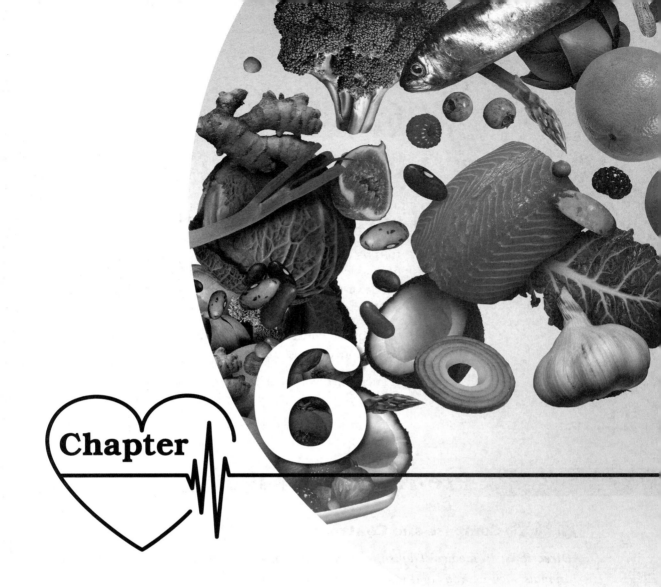

Chapter 6

Nutrition

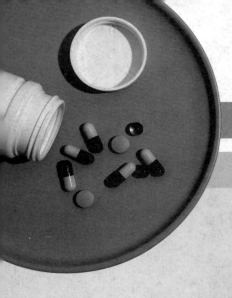

Chapter 6
Nutrition

Learning Objectives

- to master some basic skills to build medical words with affixes concerning nutrition and to expand accurate usage of amphibious words in both general and medical contexts;

- to improve comprehensive linguistic abilities to discuss issues concerning nutrition;

- to increase awareness of the importance of good nutrition to health and form a good habit of healthy eating.

Part 1　Pre-reading Tasks

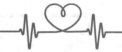

Task 1　Compare and Contrast

*Directions: In medical English, **amphibious words**, a term derived from amphibious animals such as frogs and toads that can live both on land and in water, have flexible meanings in both general contexts and medical contexts. Please consult your dictionaries, write down the Chinese equivalents of the amphibious words in the table below, and pay attention to their different meanings used as **general expressions (GE)** and **medical expressions (ME)** respectively. The first one is exemplified for you to follow.*

Amphibious Words	GE	ME
attack	袭击，攻击	（尤指常发疾病的）发作
airway		
arrest		
compound		
confusion		
course		
episode		

(Continued)

Amphibious Words	GE	ME
sign		
stroke		
tender		

Task 2 Read and Translate

Directions: Please read the following 10 pairs of sentences, and keep an eye on the 10 amphibious words you learned from the table in Task 1, which are interpreted differently as GE and ME. Translate the English sentences into Chinese.

1. All police officers are trained to defend themselves against knife <u>attacks</u>. (GE)

    _____

    _____

    People who are overweight run a risk of a heart <u>attack</u> or stroke. (ME)

    _____

    _____

2. This is the last call for passengers traveling on British <u>Airways</u> Flight 199 to Rome. (GE)

    _____

    _____

    Asthma is a chronic condition caused by inflammation of the <u>airways</u>, which can narrow them, leading to breathing difficulties. (ME)

    _____

    _____

3. The treasurer was <u>arrested</u> for trying to manipulate the company's financial records. (GE)

    _____

    _____

    Cardiac <u>arrest</u> occurs when the heart suddenly and unexpectedly stops pumping blood. (ME)

_____

_____

4. The author has conducted an exhaustive analysis of opposite compounds from the fifth edition of *Modern Chinese Dictionary*. (GE)

_____

_____

A vitamin is a chemical compound that cannot be synthesized by the human body. (ME)

_____

_____

5. When she opened the door, she was greeted by a scene of utter confusion. (GE)

_____

_____

Dizziness, mental confusion, nausea, vomiting or diarrhea also may accompany allergy. (ME)

_____

_____

6. The content of the course depends on what the students would like to study. (GE)

_____

_____

Treatment is supplemented with a course of antibiotics to kill the bacterium. (ME)

_____

_____

7. The episode underlines two things about global economic governance. (GE)

_____

_____

The freshman had suffered three <u>episodes</u> of depression within the first semester of university. (ME)

_____

_____

8. Despite <u>signs</u> of an improvement in the economy, there is no room for complacency. (GE)

_____

_____

The fever and subsequent respiratory syndrome is the most common symptom and <u>sign</u>. (ME)

_____

_____

9. Compton was sending the ball here, there, and everywhere with each <u>stroke</u>. (GE)

_____

_____

He had a minor <u>stroke</u> two years ago, which left him partly paralyzed. (ME)

_____

_____

10. Cook for a minimum of two hours, or until the meat is <u>tender</u>. (GE)

_____

_____

My scar felt very <u>tender</u>, and I dared not touch it or take a deep breath. (ME)

_____

_____

Task 3 Lead-in Questions

Directions: Read the questions below and answer them in details.

1. Text A says a healthy body requires six important nutrients, namely, carbohydrates,

proteins, fats, vitamins, minerals and water. Now there's another view claiming that one more nutrient should be added to the list. Do you know what it is? And why?

_____

_____

2. Have you heard about food therapy? Have you had an experience in which your health was improved by medicinal food?

_____

_____

3. Can you describe your daily dietary habits, and see if there's room for improvement?

_____

_____

4. Nowadays, many people, especially the elderly, would rather spend more money on health care products than take good care of their three meals a day. What do you think of this phenomenon?

_____

_____

Part 2　Texts

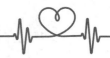

Text A

How Nutrition Plays a Role in Our Health

1　Probably most of us think health is only being **free from** illness, but it is not entirely right. For around 30 years, many national and international research organizations have focused their research on the relation of nutrition to health. Accordingly, a person should be healthy both **in terms of** physical, mental, and social well-being and not a mere absence of any disease or [1]infirmity. There is a strong relationship between nutrition and health, and we should make the right food choices to ensure we live the best life possible.

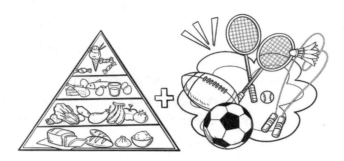

2   **WHO** announces, "Nutrition is the [2]intake of food, considered **in relation to** the body's dietary needs. Good nutrition—an adequate, well-balanced diet combined with regular physical activity—is a [3]cornerstone of good health. Poor nutrition can lead to reduced immunity, increased [4]susceptibility to disease, [5]impaired physical and mental development, and reduced [6]productivity." **Hippocrates**, the Father of medicine says, "Let food be thy medicine and medicine be thy food."

3   So, good nutrition indicates the right amount of nutrients for proper [7]utilization for achieving the highest level of health. For a healthy body, we require all these six important nutrients. [8]Carbohydrates, proteins, and fats are majorly required for bodybuilding and energy. The minerals and vitamins are required for the protection of our body and they give us resistance against the different illnesses, and they are carrying out the metabolic actions in the body and keeping the body healthy. Water is also a very important nutrient which keeps our body healthy.

4   Nutrition plays a role in promoting good health. Diets full of fruits and [9]veggies, **whole grains**, nuts, and **lean meats** have proven health benefits like lowering blood pressure, improving glucose control in [10]diabetics, weight loss, improving arthritis, and reducing the risk of cancer and cardiovascular events and so on.

5   We should also learn about the specific nutrients that can impact health. **Plant** [11]**pigments** found in bright orange and red fruits and vegetables may prevent and slow the progression of eye diseases. [12]Calcium helps to keep bones strong. Vitamin B plays a role in maintaining brain health. And [13]**flavonoids** from many plants may improve the health of our cardiovascular systems.

6   Surely you have heard this expression many times: "We are what we eat." Since we are born, we need three things to live: [14]oxygen, water, and food. Food is "fuel" through which we obtain energy and [15]compounds that help us to repair the body. Once the food is eaten, the feeding ends, and nutrition begins, which we can define as the unconscious and [16]involuntary process by which the body receives and transforms the nutritional substances that we give it through what we eat. There is no doubt that what we eat is key to achieving and maintaining optimal body function, preserving or restoring health, and protecting ourselves against future illnesses.

7 Good and balanced nutrition is very beneficial for us. Good nutrition means a portion of food that can maintain the required energy balance in our body. If we do not have the energy, we cannot perform well. For good and optimum health, we should be careful about what we are eating, how we are eating, how much we are eating, and what time we are eating.

8 The human organism has a [17]magnificent [18]resilience capacity and **adapts to** the environment that surrounds it to live **in harmony**. It can tolerate a large number of [19]pathogens or [20]**toxic agents** if the immune system is strong. However, undernutrition or overnutrition can **upset this balance**.

9 We are in an overfed and [21]paradoxically malnourished society. Currently, the food market is very large and offers us various alternatives to consume. Therefore, it is more difficult to know what we eat [22]given the reality that most processed foods come with a high [23]content of simple sugars, [24]**saturated fat**, and [25]sodium which has caused various diseases closely associated with the cardiovascular system, increasing the risk of suffering from them.

10 **Eating right** also prevents [26]obesity which is one of the main reasons for the disease. What few know is that obesity leads to other conditions such as type 2 diabetes, [27]osteoporosis, stroke, heart disease among others.

11 So, make a plan for what you eat, avoiding eating foods **loaded with** sugar, fat, and calories. The [28]culprits add extra weight to your body, weakening your bones, and making your organs work harder. They automatically **put** you **at a higher risk** for future health problems. [29]Concerning the weapon for prevention, nutrition is probably one of the most [30]valid and effective tools we have to protect our health. **Let's** make food a way to enjoy life in a healthy way.

Nishat, N. 2022. What is the relationship between nutrition and health? Theworldbook. Retrieved and adapted on August 29, 2022, from Theworldbook website.

(772 words)

Notes

1. (Para. 2) Good nutrition—an adequate, well-balanced diet combined with regular physical activity—is a cornerstone of good health. 良好的营养，即充足平衡的膳食与规律运动的配合，是健康的基石。
此句中以破折号插入的内容是对主语 good nutrition 的具体解释。

2. (Para. 3) So, good nutrition indicates the right amount of nutrients for proper utilization for achieving the highest level of health. 所以，良好的营养意味着适量的营养成分被恰当利用，以实现最高健康水平。

3. (Para. 5) flavonoids：类黄酮，泛指两个具有酚羟基的苯环通过中央三碳原子相互连接的一系列化合物。类黄酮曾被称为"维生素 P"，在生物体内的反应里，被认为具有营养功能和抗氧化或抗发炎反应功效，可以防止或减缓肿瘤的形成。类黄酮通常来自水果、蔬菜、茶、葡萄酒、植物的种子或根等。

4. (Para. 6) Once the food is eaten, the feeding ends, and nutrition begins, which we can define as the unconscious and involuntary process by which the body receives and transforms the nutritional substances that we give it through what we eat. 一旦食物被吃掉，进食结束，营养补给就开始了。我们可以把营养补给定义为身体的一种无意识、非自主的过程，在此期间身体摄入我们吃下的营养物质并将其转化。
by which... what we eat 部分包含多重从句：by which 中的 which 指代前文的 process；后面的 that 引导定语从句，表明 nutritional substances 是我们摄入体内的；through what we eat 表明我们摄入营养物质的途径是通过饮食。

5. (Para. 8) The human organism has a magnificent resilience capacity and adapts to the environment that surrounds it to live in harmony. It can tolerate a large number of pathogens or toxic agents if the immune system is strong. However, undernutrition or overnutrition can upset this balance. 人类机体具有不可思议的复原能力，能够适应周围的环境，与之和谐相处。如果免疫系统强大，它可以承受大量的病原体或有毒物质的侵袭。然而，营养不足或营养过剩会破坏这种平衡。

6. (Para. 9) Currently, the food market is very large and offers us various alternatives to consume. Therefore, it is more difficult to know what we eat given the reality that most processed foods come with a high content of simple sugars, saturated fat, and sodium which has caused various diseases closely associated with the cardiovascular system, increasing the risk of suffering from them. 目前的食品市场极为庞大，为我们提供了各种消费的选择，而且现实中大多数加工食品都带有高含量的单糖、饱和脂肪和钠，这些成分已经导致各种与心血管系统密切相关的疾病，增加了患病风险。因此，我们越来越难了解自己吃的是什么。
1）saturated fat：饱和脂肪，是由饱和脂肪酸和甘油形成的脂肪。它通常来源于动物油、肉类和奶制品等，室温下呈固体状态。椰子油、棕榈油等热带油也含有大量饱和脂肪。一般来说，饱和脂肪是必须摄取的，但饮食中比例较高的饱和脂肪酸可能会增加心血管疾病和中风的风险。

2）(be) closely associated with：与……紧密关联。

7. (Para. 10) What few know is that obesity leads to other conditions such as type 2 diabetes, osteoporosis, stroke, heart disease among others. 很少有人知道肥胖会导致其他疾病，如Ⅱ型糖尿病、骨质疏松症、中风、心脏病等。

    osteoporosis：骨质疏松症，是一种因骨质密度下降而令骨折风险增加的疾病。起因是矿物质大量流失，导致骨骼中的钙质不断流失到血液中。骨质疏松症多数情况下并不会直接导致死亡，但会增加骨折概率，极大影响患者的健康和独立生活能力。

8. (Para. 11) The culprits add extra weight to your body, weakening your bones, and making your organs work harder. 这些致病元凶给你的身体增加了额外负担，削弱了你的骨骼，并使你的器官工作更吃力。

    culprit：罪犯，元凶。此处是比喻用法，指前句所说的高糖、高脂肪等不良饮食习惯。

9. (Para. 11) Concerning the weapon for prevention, nutrition is probably one of the most valid and effective tools we have to protect our health. 说到预防武器，营养可能是我们用来保护健康最合理且最有效的工具之一。

    we have to protect our health 为定语从句，修饰前面的 tools，we 前面省略了关系代词 that/which。句尾的 to protect our health 是不定式作目的状语。

Word List

1. **infirmity** [ɪnˈfɜːrmətɪ] *n.*

    weakness or illness over a long period（长期的）体弱

2. **intake** [ˈɪnteɪk] *n.*

    the amount of food, drink, etc. that you take into your body 摄取量

3. **cornerstone** [ˈkɔːrnərstəʊn] *n.*

    the most important part of sth. that the rest depends on 基础

4. **susceptibility** [səˌseptəˈbɪlətɪ] *n.*

    the feature of being very likely to be influenced, harmed or affected by sth. 易受感染（或影响）的特性

5. **impaired** [ɪmˈperd] *adj.*

    damaged or not functioning normally 受损的

6. **productivity** [ˌprɑːdʌkˈtɪvətɪ] *n.*

    the rate of production of new biomass by an individual, population, or community 繁殖力

7. **utilization** [ˌjuːtələˈzeɪʃ(ə)n] *n.*
   the act of using 利用，使用

8. **carbohydrate** [ˌkɑːbəʊˈhaɪdreɪt] *n.*
   a substance such as sugar or starch that consists of carbon, hydrogen, and oxygen 碳水化合物

9. **veggie** [ˈvedʒɪ] *n.*
   a plant or part of a plant that is eaten as food 蔬菜

10. **diabetic** [ˌdaɪəˈbetɪk] *n.*
    a person who suffers from diabetes 糖尿病患者

11. **pigment** [ˈpɪgmənt] *n.*
    a substance that exists naturally in people, animals, and plants and gives their skin, leaves, etc. a particular color 色素

12. **calcium** [ˈkælsɪəm] *n.*
    a soft white chemical element which is found in bones and teeth, and also in limestone, chalk, and marble 钙

13. **flavonoid** [ˈfleɪvəˌnɔɪd] *n.*
    a type of substance that is found in some plants such as tomatoes, which is thought to protect against some types of cancer and heart disease 类黄酮

14. **oxygen** [ˈɑːksɪdʒ(ə)n] *n.*
    a gas that is present in air and water and is necessary for people, animals and plants to live 氧气

15. **compound** [ˈkɑːmpaʊnd] *n.*
    a substance formed by a chemical reaction of two or more elements in fixed amounts relative to each other 化合物

16. **involuntary** [ɪnˈvɑːləntəri] *adj.*
    done without conscious control 无意识的

17. **magnificent** [mægˈnɪfɪsənt] *adj.*
    very good, excellent 出色的

18. **resilience** [rɪˈzɪlɪəns] *n.*
    the ability of people or things to feel better quickly after sth. unpleasant, such as shock, injury, etc. 适应力；恢复能力

19. **pathogen** [ˈpæθədʒ(ə)n] *n.*
    a thing that causes disease 病原体

20. **toxic** ['tɑːksɪk] *adj.*
    containing poison 有毒的

21. **paradoxically** [ˌpærə'dɑːksɪklɪ] *adv.*
    in a paradoxical manner 自相矛盾地

22. **given** ['ɡɪv(ə)n] *prep.*
    when you consider sth. 考虑到，鉴于

23. **content** ['kɑːntent] *n.*
    the amount of a substance that is contained in sth. else 含量

24. **saturated** ['sætʃəreɪtɪd] *adj.*
    relating to an organic compound, especially a fatty acid, containing the maximum number of hydrogen atoms and only single bonds between the carbon atoms 饱和的

25. **sodium** ['səʊdɪəm] *n.*
    a soft silver-white metal that is found naturally only in compounds, such as salt 钠

26. **obesity** [əʊ'biːsətɪ] *n.*
    a condition characterized by the excessive accumulation and storage of fat in the body 肥胖（症）

27. **osteoporosis** [ˌɑːstɪəʊpə'rəʊsɪs] *n.*
    a condition in which the bones become weak and are easily broken, usually when people get older or because they do not eat enough of certain substances 骨质疏松症

28. **culprit** ['kʌlprɪt] *n.*
    a person or thing responsible for causing a problem 罪犯，元凶，肇事者；引发问题的事物

29. **concerning** [kən'sɜːrnɪŋ] *prep.*
    about sth. 关于

30. **valid** ['vælɪd] *adj.*
    producing the desired result; effective 有效的

Chunk List

Collocations

1. **free from** 不受……伤害；没有……的
   They long for an equal society, free from poverty and disease.
   他们向往一个没有贫穷和疾病的平等社会。

2. **in relation to** 与……相比

   The money he'd been ordered to pay was minimal in relation to his salary.

   他被要求支付的钱与他的薪水相比是极少的。

3. **whole grain** 全谷物，全麦

   Fruits, vegetables, and whole grains are rich in various nutrients.

   水果、蔬菜和全谷物富含各种营养物质。

4. **lean meat** 瘦肉

   I prefer lean meat to fatty meat.

   比起肥肉，我更喜欢瘦肉。

5. **adapt to** 适应

   We have to adapt quickly to the new system.

   我们不得不迅速适应新制度。

6. **in harmony** 融洽

   They live together in perfect harmony.

   他们十分和睦地生活在一起。

7. **upset the balance** 打破平衡

   The dam will upset the ecological balance.

   大坝会打破生态平衡。

8. **eat right** 合理饮食

   The doctor suggested that he should eat right and exercise more.

   医生建议他应该合理饮食，多运动。

9. **(be) loaded with** 富含

   The chocolate bar is loaded with fat.

   巧克力棒含有大量脂肪。

10. **put... at a high risk** 使……处于高风险中

    Heavy smokers are put at a higher risk of developing lung diseases later in their lives.

    重度吸烟者在晚年患肺病的风险更高。

Idiom and Proverb

11. **in terms of** 在……方面，从……来看

    In terms of quantity, production grew faster than ever before.

    从数量上看，生产增长的速度比以往任何时期都要快。

(Sub)Technical Chunks

12. **WHO (World Health Organization)** 世界卫生组织

About half of all smokers are killed by their addiction, WHO reported.
世界卫生组织报告说，约一半的吸烟者死于他们的烟瘾。

13. **toxic agent** 毒剂，有毒物质
They tried combining two relatively safe chemicals to produce a toxic agent.
他们试图将两种相对安全的化学物质结合起来，产生一种有毒物质。

14. **saturated fat** 饱和脂肪
Saturated fat can increase risks for heart diseases and some cancers.
饱和脂肪会增加患心脏病和某些癌症的风险。

Sentence Builder

15. **Let...** 但愿……
Let him be all right!
但愿他平安无事！

Text B

How I Learned to Manage [1]Anemia

1 I was about eight years old when I first started feeling symptoms of **iron deficiency**. Symptoms included fatigue, [2]insomnia, [3]restless legs, [4]brittle nails, cold hands and feet, [5]dizziness, pale skin, and a [6]racing heart rate. Sometimes, the anemia became [7]debilitating because the [8]exhaustion and fatigue were just so severe.

2 It took several years for me to become comfortable managing anemia.

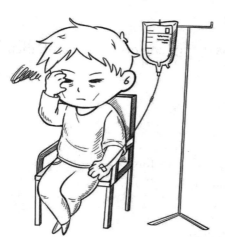

My journey included multiple diagnoses, experimenting with various treatment plans, and even surgery. With time, patience, [9]self-advocacy, and the help of loved ones, I feel I arrived at a good balance of health and happiness.

3 **It was** my mother **who** first noticed my lack of energy compared to other eight-year-olds. Most days, I would come home from school and have a nap instead of having [10]playdates with friends. My [11]frail, pale appearance [12]**blended**

in with the walls in my home. It was a clear sign that something wasn't right. My mother brought me to see our family doctor. I had blood work done which showed that my iron was significantly low, especially for someone my age. I was sent home with a [13]prescription for daily iron pills. Those iron pills **were supposed to** get me **back on my feet** and feeling like myself again, **but** that **wasn't the case**. My energy stayed low, and **over time**, other symptoms began to appear, such as severe [14]abdominal pain. My mother could tell that something was still not right.

4   About a year after my iron-deficiency diagnosis, my mother took me to a [15]gastroenterologist at a [16]pediatric hospital for **a second opinion**, along with more tests. After all the symptoms and waiting, I was diagnosed with **Crohn's disease**, an **inflammatory bowel disease**. The iron deficiency was one of several issues that **turned out to be** symptoms of Crohn's disease. Once I was diagnosed with Crohn's disease, I began proper treatment with different types of medication. My iron levels started **getting back to normal** and I started [17]thriving as a teenager.

5   By the time I reached young adulthood, I had experienced two bowel [18]resections due to Crohn's disease. Shortly after the second [19]life-altering [20]colectomy, I woke up from surgery with an [21]ostomy bag attached to my stomach to collect my waste. I started to experience [22]spells of extreme dizziness. Some days, I couldn't get out of bed because it felt like the whole room was spinning. It didn't **cross my mind** that my symptoms could possibly be related to iron deficiency. I also hadn't considered that I had lost **a large portion of** my bowel, where iron is absorbed in the body.

6   After a week of severe dizzy spells that left me lying on the bathroom floor, I contacted my doctor. To my surprise, the bloodwork revealed that my iron levels had fallen [23]tremendously. This is when my doctors told me that I was [24]anemic. They were very concerned and told me that I needed immediate medical treatment.

7   I started receiving treatments to get my iron levels back to normal. Crohn's disease was the primary cause of my iron deficiency and [25]malabsorption. With this in mind, my team of doctors decided that intravenous iron infusions would be my best treatment option. It may sound scary, but it's become part of my regular routine. At the beginning, I had to go into the infusion clinic once a week to receive them. The whole process would take about 3 to 3.5 hours. For me, the side effects included mild headaches, fatigue, and a [26]metallic taste in my mouth. It was sometimes difficult to cope, but the results over time were definitely worth it. It took about four to six weeks of weekly infusions for my body to **adjust to** treatment and to get my iron levels back to normal.

8   After some [27]trial-and-error in **figuring out** what worked for my body, I **settled on** iron infusions every three to four months. With this treatment plan, my iron levels stayed stable, no longer dropping dramatically. The new schedule not only helped to keep my energy levels up, but allowed me more time to do the things I love.

9   Ever since I started receiving regular iron infusions, it's been so much easier to manage anemia and [28]navigate through the busyness of everyday life. I enjoy a fairly busy lifestyle as a kindergarten teacher and I enjoy walking on hiking trails on the weekends. Having the energy to do the things I love is very important to me, and it finally feels like I'm able to do that.

Deveau, K. 2020. Managing anemia: What worked for me. Healthline. Retrieved and adapted on July 27, 2022, from Healthline website.

(754 words)

Notes

1. (Para. 1) restless legs：不宁腿，一般指不宁腿综合征，又称睡眠腿动症、不安腿综合征、腿不宁症候群等。临床特征是发生于下肢的一种自发的、难以忍受的痛苦的异常感觉。不宁腿以腓肠肌最为常见，大腿或上肢偶尔也会出现，通常有对称性。患者感觉在下肢深部有撕裂感、蠕动感、刺痛、烧灼感、疼痛或者瘙痒感。致病因素包括缺铁、肾功能衰竭、帕金森综合征、糖尿病、类风湿性关节炎和妊娠。一些药物治疗也会触发其症状。

2. (Para. 1) Sometimes, the anemia became debilitating because the exhaustion and fatigue were just so severe. 有时，（我的）贫血症会让我十分虚弱，因为疲劳感太强烈了。
   anemia：贫血症，是由于身体无法制造足够的血红蛋白（一种将氧气输送到血红细胞和身体各个组织的蛋白质）而造成的。患者会觉得乏力和筋疲力尽、心情忧郁和易怒不安。其他症状还包括晕厥、情感冷漠、注意力不能集中和无法忍受的寒冷感觉等。

3. (Para. 3) My frail, pale appearance blended in with the walls in my home. 我虚弱、苍白的样子几乎和我家墙壁混为一体。
   本句为比喻性说法，用白墙的颜色形容贫血症患者的面貌特征。

4. (Para. 3) My energy stayed low, and over time, other symptoms began to appear, such as severe abdominal pain. 我的精力持续低下，并且随着时间推移，还出现了严重腹痛等其他症状。

5. (Para. 4) I was diagnosed with Crohn's disease, an inflammatory bowel disease.

我被诊断为克罗恩病，一种肠道炎症性疾病。

Crohn's disease：克罗恩病，一种原因不明的肠道炎症性疾病，在胃肠道的任何部位均可发生，但多发于末端回肠和右半结肠。临床表现为腹痛、腹泻、肠梗阻，伴有发热、营养障碍等肠外表现。病程多迁延，反复发作，不易根治。许多病人出现并发症时，需进行手术治疗。复发率与病变范围、病症侵袭的强弱、病程的延长、年龄的增长等因素有关。

6. (Para. 5) Shortly after the second life-altering colectomy, I woke up from surgery with an ostomy bag attached to my stomach to collect my waste. 在第二次改变生活的结肠切除术后不久，我从手术中醒来，肚子上挂着一个收集我排泄物的造口袋。

   1）shortly after：在……之后不久。

   2）colectomy：结肠切除术，为全部或部分切除大肠的手术，常用于治疗结肠癌、结肠梗阻、结肠损伤、消化道疾病。根据术中发现结肠局部病变的位置、性质和大小，医生会选择结肠部分切除术或结肠次全切除术。

   3）ostomy bag：造口袋，造瘘袋。外科医生切除部分结肠后，可能需要进行结肠造口术（ostomy），将剩余结肠连接至体外，在腹壁开一个孔（造口），由此处将废物排出体外。结肠造瘘袋连在造口上，收集排泄物。

7. (Para. 6) After a week of severe dizzy spells that left me lying on the bathroom floor, I contacted my doctor. 在持续一周的严重间歇性眩晕让我倒在浴室地板上之后，我联系了我的医生。

   dizzy spells：间歇性眩晕，可能由脱水或低血糖、低血压等引起。轻微症状包括头晕、头痛、食欲不振、疲劳、脸色苍白、消化不良、晕车晕船等；严重症状包括直立性眩晕、四肢发冷、心悸、呼吸困难、共济失调、发音含糊，甚至昏厥，需长期卧床。

8. (Para. 7) For me, the side effects included mild headaches, fatigue, and a metallic taste in my mouth. 对我来说，（静脉铁剂输注的）副作用包括轻微头痛、疲劳，以及嘴里的金属味道。

9. (Para. 8) With this treatment plan, my iron levels stayed stable, no longer dropping dramatically. 用了这个治疗方案后，我体内的铁元素水平保持了稳定，不再急剧下降。

Word List

1. anemia [əˈnɪmɪə] *n.*
   a condition in which the blood is deficient in red blood cells, in hemoglobin, or in total volume 贫血

2. insomnia [ɪn'sɑːmnɪə] *n.*

the condition of being unable to sleep 失眠（症）

3. restless ['restləs] *adj.*

keeping moving about <u>坐立不安的</u>

4. brittle ['brɪt(ə)l] *adj.*

hard but easily broken 硬脆易碎的

5. dizziness ['dɪzɪnəs] *n.*

a sensation of spinning around and losing one's balance 眩晕

6. racing ['reɪsɪŋ] *adj.*

moving swiftly 飞快的

7. debilitating [dɪ'bɪləˌteɪtɪŋ] *adj.*

causing serious impairment of strength or ability to function 使人衰弱的

8. exhaustion [ɪg'zɔːstʃ(ə)n] *n.*

the state of being very tired 筋疲力尽

9. self-advocacy [self 'ædvəkəsɪ] *n.*

the practice of having sick or mentally handicapped people speak for themselves and control their own affairs, rather than having other people automatically assume responsibility for them 自我调适

10. playdate ['pleɪdeɪt] *n.*

a play session for small children arranged by their parents 玩耍约会

11. frail [freɪl] *adj.*

physically weak and thin 虚弱的

12. blend [blend] *v.*

to combine with sth. in an attractive or effective way 协调；融合

13. prescription [prɪ'skrɪpʃ(ə)n] *n.*

an official piece of paper on which a doctor writes the type of medicine you should have, and which enables you to get it from a chemist's shop/drugstore 处方

14. abdominal [æb'dɑːmɪn(ə)l] *adj.*

relating to or connected with the abdomen 腹部的

15. gastroenterologist [ˌgæsˌtrəʊˌentə'rɒlədʒɪst] *n.*

a physician who specializes in diseases of the gastrointestinal tract 胃肠病学家

16. pediatric [ˌpiːdɪ'ætrɪk] *adj.*

of or relating to the medical care of children 小儿科的

17. **thrive** [θraɪv] *v.*

    to grow or develop well or vigorously 茁壮成长

18. **resection** [rɪ'sekʃ(ə)n] *n.*

    excision of part of a bone, organ, or other part 切除术

19. **life-altering** [ˌlaɪf 'ɔːltərɪŋ] *adj.*

    causing to change one's life or fate 改变人生的

20. **colectomy** [kə'lektəmɪ] *n.*

    surgical removal of part or all of the colon 结肠切除术

21. **ostomy** ['ɑːstəmɪ] *n.*

    a surgical procedure that creates an artificial opening for the elimination of bodily wastes 造瘘术，造口术

22. **spell** [spel] *n.*

    a short period of time during which sth. lasts 一段时间

23. **tremendously** [trə'mendəslɪ] *adv.*

    to a great or tremendous extent 惊人地；非常地

24. **anemic** [ə'niːmɪk] *adj.*

    relating to anemia or suffering from anemia 贫血的

25. **malabsorption** [ˌmæləb'sɔːpʃ(ə)n] *n.*

    imperfect absorption of food material by the small intestines 吸收障碍

26. **metallic** [mə'tælɪk] *adj.*

    of, relating to, or resembling metal or metals 金属的

27. **trial-and-error** ['traɪəl ˌənd 'erər] *n.*

    experimenting until a solution is found 反复试验法，试错法

28. **navigate** ['nævɪɡeɪt] *v.*

    to find the right way to deal with a difficult or complicated situation 找到（对付困难或复杂情况的）正确方法

Chunk List

Collocations

1. **blend in with** 与……协调，融合

   The huts blend in perfectly with their surroundings.
   这些棚屋与周围的环境浑然一体，非常和谐。

2. **be the case** 是事实

   It is simply not the case that prison conditions are improving.

监狱条件正在改善的说法绝非事实。

3. **over time** 随着时间的推移

Ideas about the social significance of religion have changed over time.

有关宗教社会意义的观念已随时间的流逝发生了改变。

4. **a second opinion** 第二意见，其他专家的意见

I would like to see a specialist for a second opinion on my doctor's diagnosis.

针对我的医生的诊断，我想去见一位专家，听取第二意见。

5. **turn out to be** 原来是，结果是

The house they had offered us turned out to be a tiny apartment.

他们提供给我们的房子原来是一间小公寓。

6. **get back to normal** 恢复正常

Then life started to get back to normal.

后来，生活开始恢复正常。

7. **a large portion of** 一大部分

I have spent a large portion of my life here.

我已在这里度过了一生中的大部分时光。

8. **adjust to** 调整使适应

How did you adjust to college life?

你是怎么适应大学生活的?

9. **figure out** 弄明白

It took them about one month to figure out how to start the equipment.

他们用了大约一个月的时间才弄明白如何启动这台设备。

10. **settle on** 选定

Have you settled on a name for the baby yet?

你给孩子起好名字没有?

Idioms and Proverbs

11. **back on one's feet** 恢复，痊愈

Mary is back on her feet again after her operation.

玛丽手术后恢复健康了。

12. **cross one's mind** 出现在脑海中，想到

It never crossed my mind that she might lose.

我从来没想到过她会失败。

(Sub)Technical Chunks

13. **iron deficiency** 缺铁

Could iron deficiency lead to cold hands and feet?

缺铁会导致手脚冰冷吗？

14. **Crohn's disease** 克罗恩病，节段性肠炎

    Unfortunately, surgery is necessary in approximately 75% of people with Crohn's disease.

    不幸的是，大约 75% 的克罗恩病患者都需要手术治疗。

15. **inflammatory bowel disease** 炎症性肠病

    It may cause potentially severe side effects, like depression and inflammatory bowel diseases.

    它可能会引起潜在的严重副作用，比如抑郁和炎症性肠病。

Sentence Builders

16. **It is... who...** 是……（表强调）

    It was she who first introduced the pleasures of sailing to me.

    是她最先让我体会到了帆船运动的乐趣。

17. **be supposed to... but...** 本应该……但……

    He was supposed to go back to London on the last bus, but the accident prevented him.

    他本应坐最后一班公共汽车回伦敦，但这场意外拦住了他。

Part 3 **Post-reading Exercises**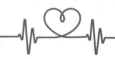

3.1 Read and Answer

3.1.1 Directions: Read Text A in Part 2 and choose the best answers to the following questions.

1. What does "health" mean according to the text?

   A. Health is only being free from illness.

   B. Health is a state of constant physical strength.

   C. Health is the absence of mental problems.

   D. Health is the good condition of physical, mental and social well-being.

2. Which of the following is true about nutrition?

   A. The more you eat, the better nutrition you get.

   B. Good nutrition is important for good health.

      C. Poor nutrition won't cause diseases.

      D. Nutrition has nothing to do with physical activity.

3. What's the negative effect of poor nutrition on one's health?

      A. Poor immunity.

      B. Increased susceptibility to disease.

      C. Damaged mental development.

      D. All of the above.

4. Which of the following is NOT an important nutrient that a healthy body needs?

      A. Carbon dioxide.   B. Fat.

      C. Mineral.   D. Water.

5. Which of the following is NOT a health benefit that a good diet has?

      A. Lowering blood pressure.

      B. Weight loss.

      C. Reducing the risk of chickenpox.

      D. Improving arthritis.

6. Which of the following statements is true about nutrients?

      A. Animal pigments may prevent eye diseases.

      B. Vitamin C is good for brain health.

      C. Calcium is good for bones.

      D. Flavonoids from plants may improve the digestive system.

7. What does the author mean by quoting "We are what we eat." in Paragraph 6?

      A. We merely need food to live.

      B. We get no energy from the food we eat.

      C. What we eat is closely related to our health.

      D. We repair compounds from the food we eat.

8. What should we pay attention to when eating?

      A. Avoid eating foods full of sugar, fat and calories.

      B. Never eat processed foods.

      C. It doesn't matter what time we eat.

      D. Never eat alternatives in the food market.

9. From which of the following sources is the text probably extracted?

      A. A biology textbook.

      B. A health magazine.

      C. A food magazine.

      D. A research paper.

10. This text is written to tell people _____.

    A. how to eat in an enjoyable way

    B. how to keep good nutrition

    C. how to prevent obesity

    D. the value of nutrition to our health

3.1.2 **Directions:** *Read Text B in Part 2 and finish the following exercises. Write T for True, F for False, or NG for Not Given in the brackets before the statements based on the instructions below.*

    True   *if the statement agrees with the claims of the author;*

    False   *if the statement contradicts the claims of the author;*

    Not Given   *if it is impossible to say what the author thinks about it.*

(   ) **1.** Anemia may make people unable to sleep well.

(   ) **2.** The author looked just the same as other 8-year-olds.

(   ) **3.** Different types of medication helped the author a lot to cope with his Crohn's disease.

(   ) **4.** Dizziness was the most obvious symptom after the author underwent the bowel surgery.

(   ) **5.** The author's iron deficiency has nothing to do with Crohn's disease.

(   ) **6.** Iron infusion caused some side effects to the author.

(   ) **7.** The fight with anemia is very difficult but effective for the author.

(   ) **8.** The author has got rid of anemia nowadays.

(   ) **9.** It was a long journey for the author to finally reach the balance of health and happiness.

(   ) **10.** The disease has a bad influence on the relationship between the author and his playmates.

3.2   Guess and Choose

Directions: *Figure out the meanings of the following medical affixes and choose the best answer from the four choices marked A, B, C and D.*

1. gluco, glycol (   )

    A. grape   B. sweetness or sugar

    C. glutton   D. glue

2. arthr, arthro (　　)
    A. artery　　　　　　B. fat　　　　　　　C. joint　　　　　　D. arteriole

3. trophy (　　)
    A. nutrition　　　　B. trolley　　　　　C. tropical　　　　D. trouble

4. gen (　　)
    A. genuine　　　　　　　　　　　　　B. gender
    C. genius　　　　　　　　　　　　　D. an agent that produces

5. hepat, hepatico, hepato (　　)
    A. heritage　　　　B. height　　　　　C. liver　　　　　　D. health

6. ost, oste, osteo (　　)
    A. oats　　　　　　B. bone　　　　　　C. oasis　　　　　　D. oath

7. oxy (　　)
    A. organ　　　　　B. ox　　　　　　　C. oxen　　　　　　D. oxygen

8. ped, pedi (　　)
    A. child　　　　　　B. aging　　　　　C. male　　　　　　D. female

9. oid (　　)
    A. oil　　　　　　　B. similar to　　　C. oily　　　　　　D. ointment

10. mal (　　)
    A. mature　　　　　B. matter　　　　　C. manual　　　　　D. wrong or bad

3.3 Read and Think

Directions: Read the following medical words built with the medical affixes from Exercise 3.2 and write down their Chinese equivalents in the table below.

Terminology	Chinese Equivalents	Terminology	Chinese Equivalents
glucose		**gluco**penia	
arthritis		**arthr**osis	
a**trophy**		hyper**trophy**	
anti**gen**		carcino**gen**	
hepatic		**hepat**itis	
osteoporosis		**osteo**arthritis	
oxygen		**ox**ide	
pediatric		**pedi**atrics	

(Continued)

Terminology	Chinese Equivalents	Terminology	Chinese Equivalents
flavon**oid**		lymph**oid**	
malnourish		**mal**absorption	

3.4 Match and Fill

3.4.1 Directions: *Match the medical terms (a–j) in the box below with their definitions (1–10).*

a. infirmity	b. osteoporosis	c. malnourished	d. nutrient
e. metabolic	f. dizziness	g. anemia	h. pediatric
i. resection	j. malabsorption		

(   ) **1.** a substance added to foods that increases their vitamin, mineral and/or protein content

(   ) **2.** a condition in which the bones become weak and are easily broken, usually when people get older or because they do not eat enough of certain substances

(   ) **3.** surgical removal of all or part of an organ, tissue, or structure

(   ) **4.** weakness; an abnormal condition of mind or body

(   ) **5.** defective or inadequate absorption of nutrients

(   ) **6.** relating to health care in children

(   ) **7.** in bad health because of a lack of food or a lack of the right type of food

(   ) **8.** an imprecise term commonly used to describe various symptoms such as faintness and imbalance

(   ) **9.** a deficiency of red blood cells

(   ) **10.** relating to a person's or animal's metabolism, the chemical processes of an organ or organism

3.4.2 Directions: *Make good use of the medical terms you learned from Exercise 3.4.1 and fill in the blanks in the sentences below. Change the form where necessary.*

1. Larger animals require more food than smaller animals, but smaller animals have a higher _____ rate.

2. Vitamin B12 is necessary to produce red blood cells and prevent _____.

3. Bones become smaller and weaker and can easily break if someone with _____ is injured.

4. Chronic diarrhea can be a sign of _____, which means nutrients are not being fully absorbed by the body.

5. Health is a state of complete physical, mental, and social well-being, not merely the absence of disease or _____.

6. Many patients surviving at least five years seem to be cured by surgical _____.

7. We eat fish, meat and beans because the _____ in them is good for our muscles.

8. Fatigue is normal, and so is _____ when you get up quickly.

9. Dr. Tom is a(n) _____ respirologist (呼吸病学专家) at the Children's Hospital of Eastern Ontario in Ottawa.

10. They have reduced their food intake, and more children are consequently _____.

3.5 Fill and Translate

3.5.1 Directions: *Choose the correct medical words from the box below to fill in the gaps (1–10) of the passage concerning food and nutrition insecurity. Change the form where necessary.*

develop	nutrition	complication	saturated	determinant
hypoglycemia	diabetes	tight	protein	veggie

Food and nutrition insecurity is a term to describe when someone is unable to access or afford enough food or enough (1) _____ food for their overall health and well-being. Food and nutrition insecurity doesn't always mean that someone goes without food; it can mean that they're not getting the healthiest kind of food. Healthy eating is an important part of managing blood sugar levels and can help prevent type 2 (2) _____. But nutritious foods can be expensive. For people who already have diabetes, buying healthy foods can compete with health care expenses for medicines, devices, and supplies.

The causes of food and nutrition insecurity are complicated. Most food and nutrition insecurity problems are related to social (3) _____ of health, such as low income or unemployment, lack of access to nutritious foods, lack of affordable housing and lack of access to health care. These causes make it hard to solve food and nutrition insecurity. The good news is that there are many programs at the national, state, and local levels that can provide food assistance.

   Nutritious foods may be too expensive for some people, which limits healthy food choices. Foods that are cheaper and easier to get tend to be lower-quality foods that are high in added sugars, (4) _____ fat, and sodium (salt). While these foods can provide plenty of calories to get someone through the day, they can also increase the risk of (5) _____ type 2 diabetes. A diet that includes plenty of vegetables, fruits, and lean (6) _____ is important for diabetes management. But some of these foods can cost more than foods that are high in calories but low in nutrition. While lower nutritional foods can cost less and provide plenty of calories, they can cause frequent spikes in blood sugar levels (hyperglycemia), which can increase the risk of diabetes-related (7) _____ like nerve damage or vision loss. Some people with diabetes may only be able to afford enough food to eat once a day, which can also make it hard to manage their diabetes. Skipping meals can increase the risk of (8) _____ (low blood sugar) and can be dangerous. With the help of food assistance programs, low-cost medicine programs, and tips on how to eat healthily on a(n) (9) _____ budget, people with diabetes can save on diabetes costs and manage it too. For example, buying frozen fruits and (10) _____, using coupons, and buying generic can help save money. It's also important to know that a diabetes care and education specialist can help people with diabetes create a meal plan that fits their lifestyle and budget.

3.5.2 Directions: Translate the underlined sentences from the passage above.

1. Food and nutrition insecurity doesn't always mean that someone goes without food; it can mean that they're not getting the healthiest kind of food.

    _____

    _____

2. The good news is that there are many programs at the national, state, and local levels that can provide food assistance.

    _____

    _____

3. But some of these foods can cost more than foods that are high in calories but low in nutrition.

    _____

    _____

4. Some people with diabetes may only be able to afford enough food to eat once a day, which can also make it hard to manage their diabetes.

_____

_____

5. It's also important to know that a diabetes care and education specialist can help people with diabetes create a meal plan that fits their lifestyle and budget.

_____

_____

3.6 Speak and Write

3.6.1 *Directions: Discuss with your group members the phenomenon described in Topic 1 below, and select a representative to report your main ideas to the class.*

Topic 1

Today people have greater awareness of staying healthy and many of them, especially the elderly, rely heavily on dietary supplements. They believe or hope that supplements can prevent or treat diseases. Bottles of supplements line the shelves at your local supermarket. These include vitamins and minerals from A to zinc. You can also find products like probiotics, herbs, and fish oil. But are they really needed for good health? And what about their risks?

3.6.2 *Directions: Discuss with your group members the phenomenon described in Topic 2 below, and write an essay in about 160 words, entitled "Natural Food and Processed Food".*

Topic 2

Traditional Chinese medicine advises people to eat the right food in the right season. More than 2,000 years ago, ancient Chinese people created an overall framework to mark the annual passage of time based on observations of the sun's movements, called "the 24 Solar Terms". The 24 Solar Terms could not only be applied to farming, but also guide the Chinese in everyday life, reminding people to adapt to changes in the seasons through suitable foods and cultural rituals. But some people prefer to enjoy all kinds of food in four seasons round. With today's technology, this has been made possible: anti-season vegetables available all year round in grocery stores, processed food with a great choice of supplements and flavors, not to mention frozen food and preserved food. Do you prefer natural food or processed food? And what are your reasons?

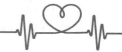

Part 4 Mini-lecture

The Categories of Chunks (Sentence Builders and Sub-technical Chunks)

Following idioms and collocations already discussed in Chapter 4, let's move on to the next two categories: sentence builders and sub-technical chunks.

Sentence builders mainly refer to sentence patterns. In "**It was** Joe **who** lent me the book", the bold-faced letters show an emphatic structure. "He was **so** fat **that** he couldn't get through the door" is an adverbial clause that indicates a result. "**Hard-working as he was**, he failed the exam" is a structure of concession. It is worth mentioning that as advanced English learners, in addition to the above-mentioned examples which you've already learned quite a lot in your primary and secondary education, you need to keep an eye on some conversation-connecting and communication-strategy chunks so as to make your linguistic output (the spoken output, in particular) more effective and successful. You may find the following examples will come in handy in online communication as they do not only connect structures and meanings but may also make up for insufficient linguistic knowledge: as a result; you know; likewise / by the same token; on the one hand... on the other hand; so to speak; in the first place / first of all; that is to say / to put it another way; in addition / on top of that / apart from that; in contrast; If we turn this the other way round...; above all; all in all / in conclusion / to sum up / in a nutshell / in a word; you know; May I have your attitude? What I mean is that... / What I want to say is that...; As I was saying earlier...

Sub-technical vocabulary is a term used to differentiate from technical vocabulary, the latter of which consists of words which are closely associated with a particular subject area. Technical vocabulary tends to be found with moderate or high frequency in a narrow range of texts, but is rarely used elsewhere. The underlined words in the following paragraph belong to the technical category as they are mostly used by a professional in a specialized area:

> "In both rheumatoid arthritis and osteoarthritis, inflammation in the joints leads to new blood vessels that release destructive enzymes. These enzymes destroy your cartilage, which causes **crippling** joint **pain**. In psoriasis, a disfiguring **skin condition**, abnormal angiogenesis under the skin helps grow the patches of raised

*red skin plaques that **are accompanied by** swelling, irritating itchiness, and **untold pain**."*[1]

Sub-technical vocabulary falls somewhere between technical vocabulary and basic words. On the one hand, they are neither items sufficiently frequent in general to be part of basic vocabulary used in day-to-day communication, nor are they tied to specific disciplines only comprehensible to professionals. To put it another way, it refers to words that are common and useful across academic disciplines which are helpful to non-professionals if they want to have a quality discussion on a specialized topic. The words in bold type in the above paragraph belong to sub-technical chunks.

Inadequate knowledge of the sub-technical category may cause problems to learners as these words are neither conspicuously frequent in the language as a whole, nor are they explicitly taught as jargons as part of a subject course. But, it is exactly an excellent grasp of sub-technical vocabulary that enables most learners of English to acquire a greater competence to articulate their viewpoints in a specialized area and therefore conduct significant and in-depth discussions or communication.

Now, we will provide you with two scenarios. First, imagine you are talking with someone about the business-running of your company, and you want to touch upon things such as hiring and firing people and going into business. Second, imagine you are having a discussion on climate change and its consequences. Think of the differences it will make, if you are equipped, or not, with an arsenal of sub-technical chunks as follows.

Sub-technical vocabulary for the first scenario: fit the job description, narrow the list down, take up references, master new skills, land a new job, be relieved of one's duties, get the sack, lose one's livelihood, be dismissed, set up a business, go into partnership with sb., make a loss, make a profit, win a contract, create jobs for, carry out market research, set a high value on customer service, sales figures, after-sales service, brisk business, booming business, annual turnover, launch a new product, strike a deal with, cut-throat competition, float the company on the stock market, go public, put in a bid for, balance the budget…

Sub-technical vocabulary for the second scenario: climatic (climate) change, weather patterns, mend our ways, searing heat, soaring temperatures, widespread flooding, catastrophic results, dire consequences, irreversible damage, irreparable

---

1 Li, W. 2019. *Eat to Beat Disease*. London: Vermillion, 11–12.

destruction, reduce one's food miles, buy local produce, offset carbon emissions, vehicle emissions, hybrid cars, alternative energy sources, renewable energy, solar heating, wind farms, geo-thermal energy, introduce green taxes, green issues, find a solution, oil supply will run dry...

You will arrive at the conclusion, we bet, that the more sub-technical vocabulary you have, the merrier.

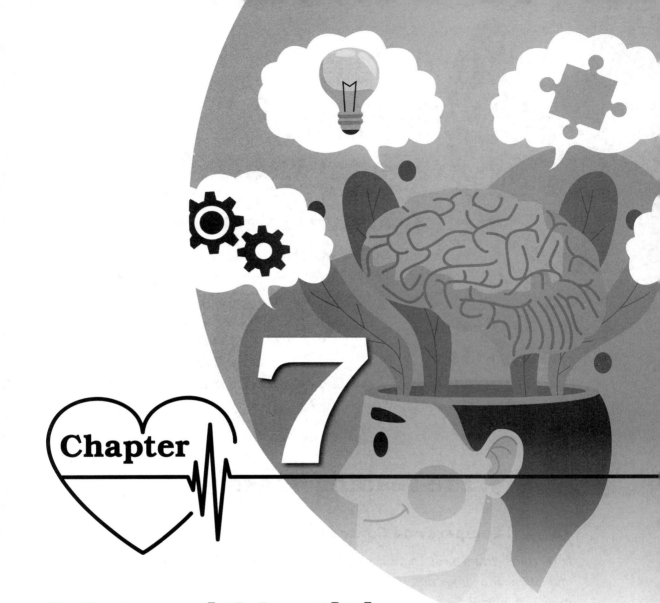

Chapter 7

Mental Health

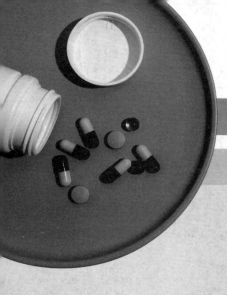

Chapter 7

Mental Health

Learning Objectives

- to master some basic skills to build medical words with affixes concerning mental health and to expand accurate usage of amphibious words in both general and medical contexts;

- to improve comprehensive linguistic abilities to discuss neurosis;

- to increase awareness of mental problems and foster a right attitude towards them.

Part 1 | Pre-reading Tasks

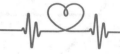

Task 1 | Compare and Contrast

Directions: In medical English, **amphibious words**, a term derived from amphibious animals such as frogs and toads that can live both on land and in water, have flexible meanings in both general contexts and medical contexts. Please consult your dictionaries, write down the Chinese equivalents of the amphibious words in the table below, and pay attention to their different meanings used as **general expressions (GE)** and **medical expressions (ME)** respectively. The first one is exemplified for you to follow.

Amphibious Words	GE	ME
depression	萧条，不景气	抑郁症，精神抑郁
disorder		
condition		
anxiety		
obsession		
withdraw		
complaint		

(Continued)

Amphibious Words	GE	ME
addictive		
remedy		
trigger		

Task 2 Read and Translate

Directions: Please read the following 10 pairs of sentences, and keep an eye on the 10 amphibious words you learned from the table in Task 1, which are interpreted differently as GE and ME. Translate the English sentences into Chinese.

1. He never forgot the hardships he witnessed during the Great Depression of the 1930s. (GE)

   _____

   _____

   Depression is closely associated with a lack of confidence and self-esteem and with an inability to express strong feelings. (ME)

   _____

   _____

2. The big question is whether increasing economic hardship will cause social unrest and political disorder. (GE)

   _____

   _____

   In this serious eating disorder, a person eats a lot of food in a short amount of time. (ME)

   _____

   _____

3. You must on no condition tell them what happened. (GE)

   _____

   _____

There is a strong possibility that the cat contracted the <u>condition</u> by eating contaminated pet food. (ME)

_____

_____

4. Many editorials express their <u>anxieties</u> about the economic chaos in the country. (GE)

_____

_____

Doctors sometimes categorize <u>anxiety</u> as an emotion or an affect depending on whether it is being described by the person having it (emotion) or by an outside observer (affect). (ME)

_____

_____

5. His <u>obsession</u> about punctuality is becoming more and more obvious. (GE)

_____

_____

Obsessive-compulsive disorder (OCD) is a type of neurosis in which an individual experiences <u>obsessions</u> or compulsions or both. (ME)

_____

_____

6. I think we should first go to the bank to <u>withdraw</u> some money for the emergency. (GE)

_____

_____

Usually an individual with neurosis should not <u>withdraw</u> the medications such as an antidepressant without medical advices. (ME)

_____

_____

7. The police officer was suspended while the <u>complaint</u> about him was investigated. (GE)

_____

_____

Much treatment, including outpatient care by clinics and medicines for many chronic <u>complaints</u>, is not covered. (ME)

_____

_____

8. In a kind of <u>addictive</u> pleasure, he watched the pink white buds of some cherry trees. (GE)

_____

_____

Unfortunately, I was diagnosed by a psychiatrist with an eating disorder and an <u>addictive</u> personality. (ME)

_____

_____

9. Especially, the economic <u>remedy</u> system and damage compensation system regarding divorce are rarely applied. (GE)

_____

_____

Aspirin is not only used for health benefits, but can be used for all kinds of unusual <u>remedies</u>. (ME)

_____

_____

10. The <u>trigger</u> for the strike was the closure of yet another factory. (GE)

_____

_____

Some causes and triggers are common to all people with depression, and some are more individual. (ME)

_____

_____

Task 3 **Lead-in Questions**

Directions: Read the questions below and answer them in details.

1. Mental health is of paramount importance as the word "health" consists of both mental and physical aspects. To your knowledge, what's the difference between neurosis and psychosis?

    _____

    _____

2. Do you know the term "OCD" and what's its full name? What, in your mind, are compulsive behaviors? If you have some personal experiences or stories about unusual, obsessive behaviors, please share with us.

    _____

    _____

3. Do you feel depressed occasionally or frequently? What usually triggers your depressive feelings? Do you have a recipe for withdrawing from those negative feelings?

    _____

    _____

4. Have you heard a nervously ill person who has been stigmatized? What's your view on the possible discrimination against the victim? In what way can you offer help to those who complain that their nerves are "in a bad way"?

    _____

    _____

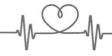

Part 2 **Texts**

Text A

OCD: The Monster in My Mind

1 Since early childhood, I have been living with a monster in my mind. To me, this is the most accurate way to describe OCD, as it feels like a separate and conflicting being that lives inside me. When I was a kid, the monster had a face but never a name. Sometimes I could have sworn I'd seen the monster shadow on my bedroom wall, [1]haunting me. But, in reality, it **left no trace** of its existence. It, and all of its weapons designed to hurt me, were simply a [2]hypochondriasis, I told myself. **It was only years later that** I learned there was a name for my suffering: [3]Obsessive [4]Compulsive Disorder.

2 My struggle with OCD started around the age of seven. Back then, it was more [5]irritating than anything. I began to feel [6]incessant urges to touch and stare at things until they felt "right", after which these compulsions helped ease the anxiety. By the time I reached ten, the obsessional side of my OCD developed [7]majorly, keeping me up all night and leading me to spend every night in the bathroom, carrying out compulsions. I had a [8]phobia of losing my hair due to the condition [9]alopecia which my mom's cousin had suffered from. I remember feeling a [10]crippling sense of anxiety in the middle of the night, when everyone else was asleep, convinced that my hair was going to **fall out**, and brushing it compulsively until I became sure that it wasn't.

3 When I started high school, things became increasingly worse. This time, my phobia became more specific. I developed a fear of hair removal cream, after hearing a horror story about it from a friend at school. Her mom's friend had accidently used the cream thinking it was shampoo, and although my friend found it [11]hilarious, I was [12]mortified. I became increasingly [13]paranoid that I unconsciously **came into contact with** hair

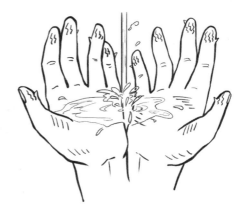

removal cream, and therefore began to participate in ""[14]cleansing compulsions" to **relieve my anxiety**. These compulsions included compulsive hand washing and the frequent spitting out of [15]saliva, both of which created difficulties in my everyday life. Because at the time, I **was** also **terrified of** the number six, I couldn't use any less than six times of soap when washing my hands, resulting in my hands to become very [16]cracked and sore, and soon attracting the attention of others. My urge to spit was a very shameful, but also very [17]addictive one for me. I did it countless times a day, even when in the most inappropriate situations, as it **relieved** so much **uneasiness and worry. In** [18]hindsight, I think this was the time in which OCD affected my life [19]outwardly the most, because my obsessions were beginning to take toll in a way that was noticeable to everyone around me. Despite this, I did not receive help. Everyone, including myself, was convinced I was just **going through an** anxious **phase**, and in a couple of years I would **grow out of** it. My mother, I learned, went through similar, although less extreme, experiences herself at my age, and never received help either. I think, **by this point**, being obsessive was just part of who I was, and nobody, not even myself, saw the point in addressing my [20]fretful way of thinking.

4　　I am now 18 years old, and finally **have a grip on** my monster. That doesn't mean it isn't there. I feel it every day, like a faded shadow threatening to [21]re-intensify. I still participate in minor [22]ritualistic compulsions in response to these thoughts, but once again to the point that is only irritating, not [23]anguishing. I still find myself struggling to control it at times, but, with a [24]mentality that at last understands. What a lot of people don't notice is that **every cloud has a silver lining**. Horrible as it is, it has its advantages when you look close enough. My obsessive personality allows me to become extremely [25]passionate and [26]driven when working on certain projects and research, which helps me **in the long term** to develop both my studies and interests. It has also taught me how to help myself when in situations that trigger anxiety, which will be helpful to me in later life, as I plan to train as a **mental health** nurse. Of course, these are just a couple of [27]minute benefits on a long list of disadvantages and difficulties, but to me, they do matter.

Townsend, L. 2016. OCD: The monster in my mind. Theocdstories. Retrieved and adapted on April 18, 2022, from Theocdstories website.

(745 words)

Notes

1. (Para.1) OCD (Obsessive Compulsive Disorder)：强迫症，属于焦虑障碍（焦虑症）的一种，是一组以强迫思维和强迫行为为主要临床表现的神经精神疾病。强迫症的特征是持续侵入的干扰性思想或形象。为缓解对这些思想或形象的焦虑，强迫症患者会出现打乱正常活动的重复性行为，尽管患者知道这样的行为不合理。重复性行为模式包括重复清洗、执行某些仪式、重复一些单词或短语，以及反复排列、接触或计数一些物体。强迫症与完美主义（perfectionism）和行为刚性（rigidity in behavior）有关，一些专家认为其与脑部神经递质 5- 羟色胺（serotonin）水平低相关。强迫症需要用行为疗法进行治疗，并使用抗抑郁药物提高脑部的 5- 羟色胺水平。

2. (Para. 1) Sometimes I could have sworn I'd seen the monster shadow on my bedroom wall, haunting me. 我敢发誓，有时就看到那魔鬼的影子出现在卧室墙上，纠缠着我。

   1）could have done 为虚拟语气，表示不确定性。

   2）haunting me 为分词结构作状语，此处表示伴随动作。分词结构作状语可以用来表示时间、原因、条件、方式、结果、让步、伴随等，此句中的逻辑主语是 monster shadow。一般情况下，逻辑主语与主句主语一致，例如：

   The boy was asleep, holding a book in his hand.（伴随动作）

   Being a hard-working young man, he was praised by the teacher.（原因）

3. (Para. 2) I began to feel incessant urges to touch and stare at things until they felt "right", after which these compulsions helped ease the anxiety. 我开始忍不住不停地摆弄一些物件，一直盯着它们直到感觉到位了，这些强迫行为帮助舒缓了焦虑情绪。

   anxiety：焦虑症，是一种伴有显著和持续的心理与身体焦虑症状的状态，且非由其他疾病造成，分为持续症状（广泛性焦虑症）与阵发症状（急性焦虑症）两类。广泛性焦虑症是指持续时间较长、无明显原因或无明确对象和内容的恐惧、紧张，并伴有植物神经症状。焦虑与恐惧情绪相近，不过恐惧是在面临危险时发生的，而焦虑发生在危险或不利情况来临之前。

4. (Para. 2) By the time I reached ten, the obsessional side of my OCD developed majorly, keeping me up all night and leading me to spend every night in the bathroom, carrying out compulsions. 到我十岁时，我的强迫症执拗的一面愈发严重，每天晚上睡不着，每晚待在浴室重复一些强迫行为。

   1）句中的 majorly 表示 seriously，其对应的形容词 major 也可表达这一含义，如 major depression（重性抑郁）。

   2）此句用到了分词结构，keeping... and leading me to... 为并列结构。

5. (Para. 2) phobia：恐惧症，是对特定物体或情景的极端持久的恐惧。恐惧的对象包括社交情景、特殊的物体（如动物或血液）或活动（如飞行或驾车穿过隧道）。恐惧症发作时常常伴有明显的焦虑和非自主神经症状，如出汗、心慌、头晕、颤抖、恶心、尿频等。英文后缀 -phobia 构成的单词表示某种恐惧症，如 acrophobia（恐高症）、agoraphobia（广场恐惧症）、claustrophobia（幽闭恐惧症）、cynophobia（恐狗症）、nyctophobia（黑暗恐惧症）。

6. (Para. 2) I remember feeling a crippling sense of anxiety in the middle of the night, when everyone else was asleep, convinced that my hair was going to fall out, and brushing it compulsively until I became sure that it wasn't. 记得半夜时分，当别人熟睡时，我会感到一阵严重焦虑，坚信我的头发要脱落了，于是忍不住梳啊梳，直到确认头发还在。

句中的 convinced that... 为过去分词从句，其逻辑主语往往能从上下文推断出，多数情况下其逻辑主语与主句主语一致，例如：

Covered with confusion, she hurriedly left the room.

7. (Para. 3) Because at the time, I was also terrified of the number six, I couldn't use any less than six times of soap when washing my hands, resulting in my hands to become very cracked and sore, and soon attracting the attention of others. 因为此时我对数字六也是感到恐惧，洗手时肥皂不擦个六次不罢休，最后洗得手皮开裂、生疼，引起旁人注意。

8. (Para. 3) I think, by this point, being obsessive was just part of who I was, and nobody, not even myself, saw the point in addressing my fretful way of thinking. 直到这时，我还是以为偏执是我性格的一部分。没有人，甚至连我自己都没有意识到我这种焦虑的思维需要治疗。

此句中的两个 point 意思不同：by this point（此时）中的 point 指某一"时刻，瞬间，阶段"；saw the point in... 中的 point 意为"意义，重要性"。

Word List

1. **haunt** [hɔːnt] *v.*
   to continue to cause problems for sb. for a long time 困扰

2. **hypochondriasis** [ˌhaɪpəkɑːnˈdraɪəsɪs] *n.*
   chronic and abnormal anxiety about imaginary symptoms and ailments 臆想症

3. **obsessive** [əbˈsesɪv] *adj.*
   (also obsessional) thinking too much about one particular person or thing, in a way that is not normal 迷恋的；难释怀的

4. **compulsive** [kəmˈpʌlsɪv] *adj.*
   (of behavior) that is difficult to stop or control 难控制的

5. **irritating** ['ɪrɪteɪtɪŋ] *adj.*

    causing irritation or annoyance 烦人的

6. **incessant** [ɪn'ses(ə)nt] *adj.*

    (usually disapproving) never stopping 持续不断的

7. **majorly** ['meɪdʒərlɪ] *adv.*

    (informal) very, extremely 非常地，极端地

8. **phobia** ['fəʊbɪə] *n.*

    a strong unreasonable fear of sth. 恐惧症

9. **alopecia** [ˌælə'piːʃə] *n.*

    loss of hair (especially on the head) 脱发（症）

10. **crippling** ['krɪplɪŋ] *adj.*

    very serious and harmful 极有害的

11. **hilarious** [hɪ'leɪrɪəs] *adj.*

    extremely funny 很滑稽的

12. **mortified** ['mɔːtɪfaɪd] *adj.*

    made to feel uncomfortable because of shame 窘迫的

13. **paranoid** ['pærənɔɪd] *adj.*

    suffering from a mental illness in which you wrongly believe that other people are trying to harm you 偏执的，妄想的

14. **cleanse** [klenz] *v.*

    to clean the skin or a wound 清洗

15. **saliva** [sə'laɪvə] *n.*

    the liquid that is produced in your mouth that helps you to swallow food 唾液

16. **cracked** [krækt] *adj.*

    damaged with lines in the surface but not completely broken 破裂的

17. **addictive** [ə'dɪktɪv] *adj.*

    (of a substance or activity) causing or likely to cause someone to become addicted to it 使人入迷的；使人上瘾的

18. **hindsight** ['haɪndsaɪt] *n.*

    the understanding of a situation or event only after it has happened or developed 事后聪明，后见之明

19. **outwardly** ['aʊtwərdlɪ] *adv.*

    on or from the outside 从外部，在外部

20. **fretful** ['fretf(ə)l] *adj.*

    behaving in a way that shows you are unhappy or uncomfortable 烦躁的，不舒适的

21. **re-intensify** [riːɪn'tensɪfaɪ] *v.*

    to increase in degree or strength again 再次加剧，再次增强

22. **ritualistic** [ˌrɪtʃʊə'lɪstɪk] *adj.*

    always done or said in the same way, especially when this is not sincere 惯常的，老套的

23. **anguish** ['æŋgwɪʃ] *v.*

    to cause to suffer extreme pain, distress, or anxiety 使……极度痛苦

24. **mentality** [men'tælətɪ] *n.*

    the particular attitude or way of thinking of a person or group 心态，思想状况

25. **passionate** ['pæʃ(ə)nət] *adj.*

    having or showing strong feelings of enthusiasm for sth. or belief in sth. 热诚的，狂热的

26. **driven** ['drɪv(ə)n] *adj.*

    (of a person) determined to succeed, and working very hard to do so 奋发努力的

27. **minute** [maɪ'nuːt] *adj.*

    small and not important 微小的，微不足道的

Chunk List

Collocations

1. **leave no trace** 不留下痕迹

   To protect environment, the travelers should leave no trace in the remote wilderness area.

   为了保护环境，旅行者应该在原野里不留痕迹。

2. **fall out**（头发、牙齿等）脱落

   Her hair started falling out as a result of radiation treatment.

   她的头发因放射治疗而开始脱落。

3. **come into contact with** 接触

   This substance should not come into contact with food.

   这种物质切莫与食物接触。

4. **relieve one's anxiety/uneasiness/worry...** 缓解某人的焦虑 / 不安 / 担忧……

   Music has been used to relieve the anxiety and elevate the spirits.

音乐已被用来缓解紧张，改善情绪。

5. **be terrified of** 惧怕

   He was terrified of spiders.

   他惧怕蜘蛛。

6. **in hindsight** 回想

   My friends and family members thought I had gone mad and, in hindsight, they were quite right.

   我的朋友和家人都曾认为我疯了，回想起来，他们都是对的。

7. **go through a(n)... phase** 经历……阶段

   Once you go through a Romeo-Juliet phase of a relationship, you can become desperate.

   一旦你经历过一段罗密欧与朱丽叶般的恋情，你就会变得绝望。

8. **grow out of** 因长大或改变而不再有（某行为、兴趣等）

   Most children who wet their beds eventually grow out of it.

   大部分小时候尿床的孩子，长大以后就好了。

9. **by this point** 目前为止

   He was a great king before, but by this point has become a weak man.

   他曾经是王者，但此时此刻却变成了弱者。

10. **have a grip on** 控制

    No one seems to have a firm grip on the company at the moment.

    这时候，好像没有人能够牢牢地掌控公司。

11. **in the long term** 长期

    A healthy lifestyle will have very positive results in the long term.

    健康的生活方式从长远来看将产生非常积极的效果。

Idiom and Proverb

12. **every cloud has a silver lining** 黑暗中总有一线光明

    As they say, every cloud has a silver lining. We have drawn lessons from the decisions taken.

    正如他们所说，黑暗中总有一线光明。我们已从所做的决定中汲取了教训。

(Sub)Technical Chunks

13. **OCD (Obsessive Compulsive Disorder)** 强迫症

    They warn that heavy dependence on microblogs can lead to mental problems like anxiety disorder or OCD.

    他们警告称，对微博高度依赖可能导致像焦虑症或强迫症这样的精神问题。

14. **mental health** 心理健康

On the individual level, exercise can improve both our physical and mental health.

对于每个人来说，锻炼可以改善我们的身体和心理健康。

Sentence Builder

15. **It was only years later that...** 多年之后，终于……

It was only years later that he developed a sense of gratitude for the strangers' help.

多年之后，他终于对陌生人的帮助心存感激。

Text B

Helping Someone with Depression

1   Depression is a serious but treatable disorder that affects millions of people, from the young to the old and from **all walks of life**. It **gets in the way** of everyday life, causing tremendous pain, hurting the sufferers and impacting everyone around them. Your support and encouragement can play an important role in your loved one's recovery. Here's how to **make a difference**.

2   Start by learning all you can about depression. Symptoms include poor appetite or significant weight loss, **sleeping disturbance** (insomnia, for example), loss of interest in ¹stimulating activities, ²**psychomotor** ³**agitation or** ⁴**retardation**, low ⁵self-esteem, self-defeating thinking, and recurrent thoughts of suicide. Four or five of the above symptoms, occurring nearly every day for at least two weeks, ⁶constitute **major depression**.

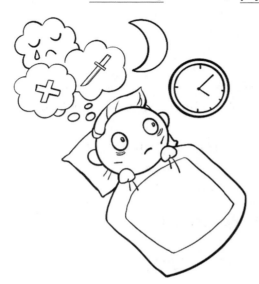

3   If someone you love is depressed, you may experience a number of difficult emotions, including helplessness, frustration, anger, fear, guilt, and sadness. These feelings are all normal. It's not easy dealing with a ⁷depressive. And if you neglect your own health, it can become ⁸overwhelming. As you **reach out**, don't forget to look after your own emotional health—you'll need it to provide the full support your loved one needs.

4   Your [9]companionship and support can be crucial to one's recovery. You can help them cope with depression symptoms, **overcome negative thoughts**, and **recharge their batteries**. But sometimes it is hard to know what to say when speaking to someone about depression. When faced with your worries, the depressive may get angry, feel [10]insulted, or ignore your concerns. You may be unsure what questions to ask or how to be supportive.

5   If you don't know where to start, remember that being a compassionate listener is much more important than giving advice. You don't have to try to "fix" your friend or family member; you just have to be a good listener. Often, the simple act of talking face to face can be an enormous help to someone suffering from depression. Encourage the depressed persons to talk about their feelings, and listen **without judgment**.

6   Don't expect a single conversation to **work wonders**. Depressed people tend to **withdraw from** others and [11]isolate themselves. You may need to express your concern and willingness to listen over and over again. Be gentle, yet [12]persistent.

7   Finding a way to start a conversation about depression with your loved one is always the hardest part. You could try saying:

- "I have been feeling concerned about you lately."
- "Recently, I have noticed some differences in you and wondered how you are doing."
- "I wanted to **check in with** you because you have seemed pretty [13]down lately."

8   Once you are talking, you can ask questions such as:

- "When did you begin feeling like this?"
- "Did something happen that made you start feeling this way?"
- "How can I best support you right now?"
- "Have you thought about getting help?"

9   Remember, being supportive involves offering encouragement and hope. Very often, this is a matter of talking to the persons in language that they will understand and can respond to while in a depressed state of mind.

10   What you can say also matters. Better say:

- "You're not alone. I'm here with you waiting for the **light at the end of the tunnel**."
- "It may be hard to believe right now, but the way you're feeling will change."
- "You're important to me. Your life is important to me."

11 Avoid saying:

- "Everyone goes through tough times."
- "Try to **look on the bright side**."
- "Just **snap out of it**."

12 While you can't control someone else's recovery from depression, you can encourage them to seek help. Getting a depressed person into treatment can be difficult. Depression [14]saps energy and [15]motivation, so even the act of making an appointment or finding a doctor can seem [16]daunting to your loved one. Depression also involves negative ways of thinking. The depressed person may believe that the situation is hopeless and treatment pointless.

13 If your friend or family member resists getting help, suggest a general check-up with a physician. Your loved one may be less anxious about seeing a family doctor than a mental health professional. A regular doctor's visit is actually a great option, since the doctor can **rule out** medical causes of depression. If the doctor diagnoses depression, he/she can refer your loved one to a [17]psychiatrist or [18]psychologist. Sometimes, this "professional" opinion makes all the difference.

14 Offer to help the depressed persons find a doctor or [19]therapist and go with them on the first visit. Finding the right treatment provider can be difficult, and is often a trial-and-error process. For a depressed person already low on energy, it is a huge help to have assistance making calls and looking into the options.

Smith, M., Robinson, L. & Segal, J. 2022. Helping someone with depression. Helpguide.
Retrieved and adapted on September 22, 2022, from Helpguide website.

(778 words)

Notes

1. (Para. 2) psychomotor agitation or retardation：精神运动性激越或迟滞。前者指病人脑中反复思考一些没有目的的事情，思维内容无条理，大脑持续处于紧张状态，无法进行创造性思考，在行为上则表现为烦躁不安。有时候，患者会不能控制自己的行为，但是又不知道自己为何烦躁，因此患者可能会惶惶不可终日，临床上易被误诊为焦虑症。与之相反，精神运动性迟滞则表现为大脑思维贫乏、迟钝；在心理上表现为思维发动的迟缓，在行为上表现为显著持久的意志行为迟缓。

2. (Para. 2) Four or five of the above symptoms, occurring nearly every day for at least two weeks, constitute major depression.（如果）以上症状的四至五种几乎每天出现并持续两周以上，则视为重度抑郁。

   1）occurring... two weeks 为分词短语，作 symptoms 的主语补足语。

   2）major depression：重性抑郁障，也被称为重度抑郁或临床抑郁症。特征是持续性地情绪低落、丧失生趣。重性抑郁发作期是指在两周或更长时间里，患者持续地经历绝望感、丧失生活乐趣、精力衰竭，产生自杀想法等。

3. (Para. 3) As you reach out, don't forget to look after your own emotional health—you'll need it to provide the full support your loved one needs. 当你伸出援手时，别忘记照顾你自己的情绪（心理）健康 —— 你需要它来为你珍爱的人提供所需的全力支持。

   1）it 指代 your own emotional health。

   2）后半句中，to provide... needs 为动词不定式作目的状语；your loved one needs 是修饰 the full support 的定语从句。

4. (Para. 4) You can help them cope with depression symptoms, overcome negative thoughts, and recharge their batteries. 你可以帮助他们应对抑郁症状，克服消极的想法，令他们重新充满活力。

   1）cope with：处理，应对。

   2）recharge their batteries 为比喻说法，本意为"重新给他们的电池充电"，此处意为"让抑郁的人重新充满活力"。

5. (Para. 5) Often, the simple act of talking face to face can be an enormous help to someone suffering from depression. 通常来说，简单的面对面谈话对遭受抑郁之苦的人而言是一个极大的帮助。

6. (Para. 7) Finding a way to start a conversation about depression with your loved one is always the hardest part. 如何与你珍爱的人开始谈论抑郁症，这总是最难的部分。

7. (Para. 12) Depression saps energy and motivation, so even the act of making an appointment or finding a doctor can seem daunting to your loved one. 抑郁症使人精力衰竭，动机受挫，所以即使是预约诊断或求医也可能会令你所珍爱的人退缩。

8. (Para. 13) psychiatrist：精神病学家，精神科医生。他们以精神医学为专业，对人体作为一种有机体及其神经功能有充分了解，其治疗方法依赖生物学概念和研究数据。精神科医生可以对患者进行体格检查及心理治疗，具有处方资格，可以使用药物治疗患者。

9. (Para. 13) psychologist：心理学家，心理咨询师。他们为有心理障碍 [包括焦虑、沮丧、愤怒、成瘾、创伤后精神紧张障碍（PTSD）、多动症（ADHD）或家庭问题等] 的患者提供心理或行为干预。心理咨询师通常没有处方资格，但如果获得认证，也可以开具处方。

Word List

1. **stimulating** ['stɪmjʊleɪtɪŋ] *adj.*
   making people feel enthusiastic 使人兴奋的

2. **psychomotor** [ˌsaɪkəʊ'məʊtər] *adj.*
   of, relating to, or characterizing movements of the body associated with mental activity 精神运动的

3. **agitation** [ˌædʒɪ'teɪʃ(ə)n] *n.*
   a state of anxiety or nervous excitement 焦虑；紧张激动

4. **retardation** [ˌriːtɑːr'deɪʃ(ə)n] *n.*
   abnormal slowness of thought or action 延迟，阻滞

5. **self-esteem** [ˌself ɪ'stiːm] *n.*
   a feeling of being happy with your own character and abilities 自尊（心）

6. **constitute** ['kɑːnstɪtuːt] *v.*
   (not used in the progressive tenses) to be considered to be sth. 被视为（不用于进行时）

7. **depressive** [dɪ'presɪv] *n.*
   a person who is suffering from the medical condition of depression 抑郁症患者

8. **overwhelming** [ˌəʊvər'welmɪŋ] *adj.*
   affecting you so strongly that you do not know how to deal with it 令人难以应对的

9. **companionship** [kəm'pænjənʃɪp] *n.*
   the pleasant feeling that you have when you have a friendly relationship with sb. and are not alone 友情

10. **insult** [ɪn'sʌlt] *v.*
    to say or do sth. that offends sb. 侮辱，冒犯

11. **isolate** ['aɪsəleɪt] *v.*
    to separate sb./sth. physically or socially from other people or things（使……）孤立，隔离

12. **persistent** [pər'sɪstənt] *adj.*
    determined to do sth. despite difficulties, especially when other people are against you and think that you are being annoying or unreasonable 坚持不懈的

13. **down** [daʊn] *adj.*

    (informal) sad or depressed 悲伤的，情绪低落的

14. **sap** [sæp] *v.*

    to weaken or destroy sth. gradually 削弱，逐渐破坏

15. **motivation** [ˌməʊtɪˈveɪʃ(ə)n] *n.*

    the reason or reasons one has for acting or behaving in a particular way 动机；
    动力

16. **daunting** [ˈdɔːntɪŋ] *adj.*

    seeming difficult or intimidating to deal with in prospect 看上去棘手的，使人畏
    惧的

17. **psychiatrist** [saɪˈkaɪətrɪst] *n.*

    a doctor who studies and treats mental illnesses 精神科医生

18. **psychologist** [saɪˈkɑːlədʒɪst] *n.*

    a scientist who studies and is trained in psychology 心理学家

19. **therapist** [ˈθerəpɪst] *n.*

    a person who is skilled in a particular type of therapy, especially psychotherapy
    （尤指心理疗法的）治疗师

Chunk List

Collocations

1. **get in the way** 妨碍，阻碍

    He wouldn't allow emotions to get in the way of him doing his job.
    他不会让情绪妨碍自己的工作。

2. **make a difference** 有影响，有关系

    Changing schools made a big difference to my life.
    转学对我的一生有着重大影响。

3. **reach out** 提供援助

    The church needs to find new ways of reaching out to young people.
    教会需要寻找新途径来为年轻人提供帮助。

4. **overcome negative thoughts** 克服消极思想

    The way to overcome negative thoughts is to develop opposing, positive emotions
    that are stronger and more powerful.
    克服消极思想的方法是产生与之对立的、更为强大有力的积极情绪。

5. **without judgment** 不作评判

She gave advice carefully and without judgment.
她提建议时很谨慎，而且不妄加评判。

6. **withdraw from** 脱离，不与人交往

Some people withdraw from friends and family.
有些人会脱离朋友与家庭。

7. **check in with** 与……联系

If you experience any of the following symptoms, check in with your physician.
如果你有下列任何症状，请和你的医生联系。

8. **rule out** 排除

Police have not ruled out the possibility that the man was murdered.
警方尚未排除那个男子是被谋杀的可能性。

Idioms and Proverbs

9. **all walks of life** 各行各业

One of the greatest pleasures of this job is meeting people from all walks of life.
这份工作最大的乐趣之一就是结识来自各行各业的人。

10. **recharge one's batteries** 养精蓄锐，休整

He wanted to recharge his batteries and come back feeling fresh and positive.
他想去休整一下，然后回来时精力充沛、积极向上。

11. **work wonders** 创造奇迹，产生奇效

A few moments of relaxation can work wonders.
短暂的放松能产生奇效。

12. **light at the end of the tunnel** 曙光，希望

After four-year work on the project, we're beginning to see the light at the end of the tunnel.
这个项目我们搞了四年，现在总算开始看到希望了。

13. **look on the bright side** 看到光明的一面，保持乐观

By training yourself to look on the bright side, you will gain more courage to face difficulties.
通过训练自己保持乐观（的态度），你会获得更多的勇气以面对困难。

14. **snap out of it** 抛掉不愉快的情绪，振作起来

You've been depressed for weeks. It's time you snap out of it.
你情绪低落好几周了，现在该振作起来了。

(Sub)Technical Chunks

15. **sleeping disturbance** 睡眠障碍

The most common symptoms included difficulty in falling asleep and sleeping disturbance.

入睡困难和睡眠障碍是最常见的症状。

16. **psychomotor agitation or retardation** 精神运动性激越或迟滞

    People with psychomotor agitation experience excessive movement and thought. On the contrary, people suffering from psychomotor retardation usually have unaccountable difficulty in carrying out some "automatic" self-care tasks, as it may take more than an hour to dress oneself in the morning.

    精神运动性激越的病人行动或思维过于激动。相反，精神运动性迟滞的病人则往往难以完成一些本可以"自动"完成的自理行为，比如早上穿衣服可能会耗时一小时以上。

17. **major depression** 重性抑郁

    Surprisingly, crying is more commonly associated with minor forms of depression than with major depression involving suicidal thoughts.

    令人惊讶的是，哭泣更多地与轻度抑郁症联系在一起，而不是与有自杀念头的重度抑郁症相关。

Part 3 Post-reading Exercises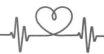

3.1 Read and Answer

3.1.1 Directions: *Read Text A in Part 2 and choose the best answers to the following questions.*

1. What does "monster" refer to in the text?

   A. A kind of horrible beast.

   B. The shadow of an animal.

   C. The fear of losing hair.

   D. A kind of mental disorder.

2. Which of the following is NOT a symptom of the author's OCD?

   A. Persistent addiction to drugs.

   B. A strong restless desire to touch and stare at things.

   C. Poor sleep.

   D. The recurrent phobia of losing her hair.

3. Why didn't the author receive any help during her fight with OCD?

A. Because it's nothing serious.

B. Because she would grow out of it finally.

C. Because no one was aware of the severity of the problem.

D. Because no one liked her.

4. Which of the following is true according to the text?

A. The author knew clearly what the "monster" actually was in her early childhood.

B. The author got kind of anxiety and phobia after getting OCD.

C. The author got some help from friends around her.

D. The author finally got rid of OCD.

5. From Paragraph 3 we can infer that _____.

A. people are often unaware of the fact that OCD is a disease at first

B. everyone began to notice the author's behavior

C. the author's mother also had OCD

D. OCD is not a big problem

6. What advantage did OCD bring to the author?

A. She became very friendly in her life.

B. She became very helpful to other people.

C. She got to know the importance of working hard.

D. She got to know how to help herself in anxious situations.

7. When struggling with OCD, the author experienced the following feelings EXCEPT _____.

A. anxiety   B. fear

C. indifference   D. compulsion

8. This text would most likely be found in a book of _____.

A. entertainment   B. novel

C. clinical cases   D. history

9. The author's attitude toward her OCD in the end is _____.

A. terrified   B. negative

C. critical   D. positive

10. What is the main idea of this text?

A. The author didn't fight against anxiety.

B. The author had been struggling with OCD during her growth.

C. How the author overcame her phobia.

D. How the author learned to avoid growing problems.

3.1.2 ***Directions:*** *Read Text B in Part 2 and finish the following exercises. Write T for True, F for False, or NG for Not Given in the brackets before the statements based on the instructions below.*

> *True*   *if the statement agrees with the claims of the author;*
>
> *False*   *if the statement contradicts the claims of the author;*
>
> *Not Given*   *if it is impossible to say what the author thinks about it.*

(   ) 1. Depression is a mental disorder that only causes psychological symptoms.

(   ) 2. To help someone in depression, you can try to be a good listener first.

(   ) 3. If you are not a doctor, you can do nothing to help someone with depression symptoms.

(   ) 4. Depressed people are supposed to visit their family doctors once a week.

(   ) 5. A depressed person may refuse the help from others.

(   ) 6. Symptoms of depression include sleeping disturbance, loss of interest in stimulating activities, high self-esteem, recurrent thoughts of suicide, etc.

(   ) 7. A doctor can rule out conditions that may cause depression with a physical examination, a personal interview, and lab tests.

(   ) 8. Persuading a depressed person to be optimistic can make him/her feel better.

(   ) 9. You should take care of your own emotional health when helping others in depression.

(   ) 10. More than one kind of difficult emotions may appear in a depressed person.

3.2 **Guess and Choose**

Directions: *Figure out the meanings of the following medical affixes and choose the best answer from the four choices marked A, B, C and D.*

1. psycho, psych (   )
   A. head   B. brain   C. mind   D. organ

2. encephalo, encephal, cephalo, cephal (   )
   A. brain   B. soul   C. neck   D. forehead

3. cerebro, cerebr (   )
   A. cell   B. tissue   C. head   D. ear

4. neuro, neur (　　)
  A. spirit　　　　B. nerve　　　　C. back　　　　D. arm

5. dia (　　)
  A. mild　　　　B. slight　　　　C. moderate　　　　D. complete

6. gnoso, gnos, gnosis (　　)
  A. sight　　　　B. knowledge　　　　C. hearing　　　　D. sensation

7. patho, path, pathy (　　)
  A. illness　　　　B. pain　　　　C. breath　　　　D. cough

8. algia (　　)
  A. anger　　　　B. burning　　　　C. ache　　　　D. dizziness

9. tox (　　)
  A. top　　　　B. touch　　　　C. toll　　　　D. poison

10. phobia (　　)
  A. photo　　　　B. fear　　　　C. happiness　　　　D. sadness

3.3 Read and Think

Directions: Read the following medical words built with the medical affixes from Exercise 3.2 and write down their Chinese equivalents in the table below.

Terminology	Chinese Equivalents	Terminology	Chinese Equivalents
psychology		**psychi**atrist	
electro**encephalo**gram (EEG)		**encephalo**pathy	
pathology		psycho**path**	
cerebral		**cerebr**um	
diagnose		**diagnosis**	
neurosis		**neuro**transmitter	
neur**algia**		arthr**algia**	
toxin		in**tox**ication	
zoo**phobia**		photo**phobia**	
hydro**phobia**		astra**phobia**	

3.4 Match and Fill

3.4.1 Directions: *Match the medical terms (a–j) in the box below with their definitions (1–10).*

a. insomnia	b. retardation	c. psychiatrist	d. therapist
e. physician	f. recurrent	g. persistent	h. paranoid
i. alopecia	j. hypochondriasis		

(   ) **1.** a medical doctor specialized in mental disorders

(   ) **2.** a practitioner of medicine, as contrasted with a surgeon

(   ) **3.** the condition of being delayed or impeded

(   ) **4.** existing or remaining in the same state for an indefinitely long time

(   ) **5.** exhibiting or characterized by irrational distrust or suspicion of others

(   ) **6.** suffering from a condition of hair loss

(   ) **7.** a mental disorder characterized by excessive fear of or preoccupation with a serious illness, despite medical testing and reassurance to the contrary

(   ) **8.** denoting the symptoms occurring or appearing again or repeatedly

(   ) **9.** the inability to obtain an adequate amount or quality of sleep

(   ) **10.** a person providing or conducting any form of medical or psychological treatment

3.4.2 Directions: *Make good use of the medical terms you learned from Exercise 3.4.1 and fill in the blanks in the sentences below. Change the form where necessary.*

1. They are inherently jealous and suspicious, often _____ about the relationship.

2. The horror movie overwhelmed him so much that he began to suffer from a sleeping disorder, even _____.

3. Sensitive and introverted, the suspicious person developed obstacle of _____.

4. The teenager complains of premature cases of _____ and more typical male pattern baldness.

5. Most growth _____ occurs by the age of two and is irreversible.

6. They told me it was an anxiety attack of some sort, and referred me to a(n) _____ for further assessment.

7. After training I often go and do some extra strength training or get a treatment from the physical _____ and a massage.

8. A(n) _____ cannot become a specialist in heart surgery, obstetrics, and psychiatry.

9. He said the research offers the first direct proof that the virus causes _____ infection in blood vessels.

10. As you can see, before the treatment, there were multiple, _____ tumors in his liver.

3.5 Fill and Translate

3.5.1 Directions: *Choose the correct medical words from the box below to fill in the gaps (1–10) of the passage concerning mental illnesses. Change the form where necessary.*

clinic	therapy	persistence	disorder	anxiety
obsessive	condition	severe	depression	complain

Mental illnesses are health (1) _____ involving changes in emotion, thinking or behavior or a combination of these. Mental illnesses are associated with distress or problems functioning in social, work or family activities. Mental illnesses include many different conditions that vary in degree of (2) _____, ranging from mild to moderate to severe. Depression or major (3) _____ disorder is a common and serious medical illness that negatively affects how you feel, the way you think and how you act. Depression causes feelings of sadness or a loss of interest in activities once enjoyed. Depression can be long-lasting or recurrent, and it can lead to a variety of emotional and physical (4) _____ and decrease a person's ability to function at work and at home. Obsessive Compulsive Disorder is a disorder in which people have recurring, unwanted thoughts, ideas or (5) _____ that make them feel driven to do something repetitively. The repetitive behaviors, such as hand washing, checking on things or cleaning, can significantly interfere with a person's daily activities and social interactions. (6) _____ disorders differ from normal feelings of nervousness or anxiousness, and involve excessive fear. Anxiety disorders are the most common of mental disorders and affect nearly 30 percent of adults at some point in their lives. Personality (7) _____ are long-term patterns of behavior and inner experiences that differs significantly from what is expected. The pattern of experience and behavior begins by late adolescence or early adulthood and causes distress or problems in functioning. Without treatment, personality disorders can be (8) _____. Mental illness is nothing to be ashamed of. It is a medical problem, just like heart disease or diabetes.

If you or someone you know has a mental disorder, is struggling emotionally, or has concerns about their mental health, there are ways to get help. Treatment for mental illnesses usually consists of (9) _____, medication, or a combination of the two. The sufferers can be effectively treated with talking therapies, such as cognitive behavior therapy or psychotherapy. Antidepressants can be an effective form of medication for moderate to severe depression but are not the first line of treatment for cases of mild depression. Physical exercise is recommended for management of mild depression, and has a moderate effect on symptoms. What's more, (10) _____ trials are research studies that look at new ways to prevent, detect, or treat diseases and conditions, including mental illnesses. The goal of clinical trials is to determine if a new test or treatment works and is safe.

3.5.2 **Directions:** *Translate the underlined sentences from the passage above.*

1. Mental illnesses are associated with distress or problems functioning in social, work or family activities.

    _____

    _____

2. Depression causes feelings of sadness or a loss of interest in activities once enjoyed.

    _____

    _____

3. The repetitive behaviors, such as hand washing, checking on things or cleaning, can significantly interfere with a person's daily activities and social interactions.

    _____

    _____

4. The pattern of experience and behavior begins by late adolescence or early adulthood and causes distress or problems in functioning.

    _____

    _____

5. Antidepressants can be an effective form of medication for moderate to severe depression but are not the first line of treatment for cases of mild depression.

    _____

    _____

3.6 Speak and Write

3.6.1 **Directions:** *Discuss with your group members the phenomenon described in Topic 1 and Topic 2 below, and select a representative to report your main ideas to the class.*

Topic 1

People with Obsessive Compulsive Disorder are typically aware of their behaviors. Some see such obsessive behaviors as advantages that can make them extremely passionate when working on a project. On the other hand, people with addictions are often unaware of or unconcerned about the negative consequences of their actions. They think it is overexaggerating to treat such compulsions as a disease. What is your view?

Topic 2

People with the compulsive hoarding syndrome gather many objects such as newspapers, clothing, food and even animals, and seemingly cannot remove them. Hoarders believe the objects could be useful some day and it is a way to save resources. They may even develop an emotional connection to such things. However, it is worried that it may endanger their physical health when hoarders live with so much clutter. Severe health risks can also result from collecting waste, food or materials that can cause fires. What is your view on compulsive hoarding?

3.6.2 **Directions:** *Write an essay in about 160 words, entitled "Is It Possible for Individuals to Avoid the Occurrence of Mental Illnesses?". Think about how you can develop more supporting details to convince others of your arguments or counter-arguments. The following statements are respectively presented as references for you.*

Arguments for:

- Those with a family history of mental illnesses usually screen the disorder in early childhood, and thus they are consciously to avoid the problem.

- Some therapies and medications are very effective treatment to control the mental illnesses.

- Some mild depression, obsessions and anxiousness can be alleviated through physical exercise and won't significantly affect their family, work and social interactions.

  …

Arguments against:

- Mental illnesses mean persistent and recurrent struggles for the sufferers in their whole life.

- Medications such as antidepressants have many side effects which make individuals' physical health deteriorate and trigger many medical problems.

- Mental disorders can not be cured and people with mental complaints are frequently stigmatized as crazy and insane psychos.

...

Part 4   Mini-lecture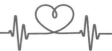

How to Group Chunks in a Vocabulary Notebook

It's already suggested that we need to make a point of writing down the useful chunks we come across in reading and listening. Next, let's discuss a technical part of this writing job: How to organize the chunks into our vocabulary notebooks? Of course, the easiest, or the most "natural" way we can think of, is to write down the chunks one by one in line with the sequence we meet them. But, we may get a very "messy" chunk list in terms of a variety of meanings the different chunks offer. After all, chunks with multifarious meanings "scattered", so to speak, in a notebook, will cause inconvenience when we want to retrieve them in real communication. Besides, if we hope to commit the chunks to memory more effectively and efficiently, we'd better seek a tidier way of organization.

Grouping chunks by meaning is a useful method. If we divide our notebooks into broad sections, and group together the chunks which share similar meanings or are related to one specific topic, it not only helps us remember the chunks longer but also improves our access to them for real use. Therefore, we need to first choose the topics and then write down the chunks whose meanings are related to a specific topic on the right pages of the notebook. For example, if we name "environment" as a topic, we can therefore put into this section chunks such as "greenhouse effect" "global warming" "rising sea levels" "shrinking habitats" "carbon emissions" "reduce our carbon footprints" "greenhouse effect" "green taxes" "pristine environments" "household wastes" "destruction of the ozone layer" "alternative energy" "piecemeal conservation", etc.

Of course, to decide how many topics will be included in a notebook is an individual behavior so long as the division and grouping make sense to the writer personally. Meanwhile, we may find that a particular chunk can be grouped into different sections, as it fits more than one topic. We can also provide an example for each chunk if we want to familiarize ourselves with its use. Let's illustrate more clearly this method with a topic named "emotions and feelings" whose components are chunks describing different moods and feelings. It's a good idea if we view these chunks as an extension to what we have already learned, as both depressives and obsessives are prone to more exaggerated moods and feelings compared with the normal. A topic can be further divided to several sub-categories depending on personal preferences. As we can see in the following examples, the topic of emotions and feelings includes joy and happiness, uneasiness and sadness, anger, and other feelings.

Topic: Emotions and Feelings

1. Joy and Happiness

1) *jump for joy*

- Angie *jumped for joy* when she knew her ill-tempered manager was transferred to another department.

2) *on top of the world*

3) *have a barrel of fun*

4) *get a kick out of*

5) *on cloud nine*

6) *to one's heart's content*

7) *feast one's eyes on*

…

2. Uneasiness and Sadness

1) *have the jitters*

- Tom is very likely to *have the jitters* when faced with a crowd of people in public.

2) *on pins and needles*

3) *have butterflies in one's stomach*

4) *get on one's nerves*

5) *drive someone up the wall*

6) *down in the dumps*

7) *get one's back up*

...

3. Anger

1) *fly into a rage*

   • He almost *flew into a rage* and kept telling me it's none of my business.

2) *fly off the handle*

3) *blow one's lid*

4) *make one's blood boil*

5) *get one's goat*

6) *drive one round the bend*

7) *bad blood*

...

4. Other Feelings

1) *feel like a square peg in a round hole*

   • In the very beginning, you may *feel like a square peg in a round hole* in your new job.

2) *feel like a fish out of water*

3) *out of one's element*

4) *feel at a loss*

5) *sick and tired of*

6) *give one goose bumps*

7) *feel a lump in one's throat*

8) *take one's breath away*

9) *blow one's mind*

...

Remember to leave enough space (pages) for each section, and we may prepare several notebooks instead of one to work on.

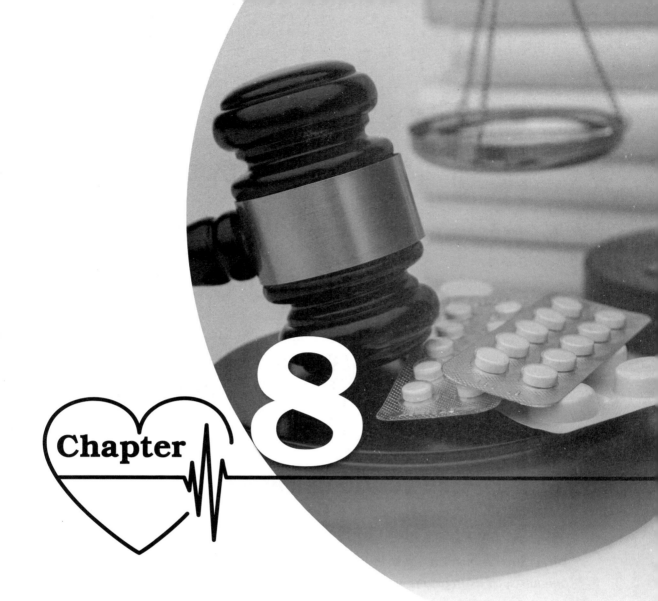

Chapter

8

Medical Ethics

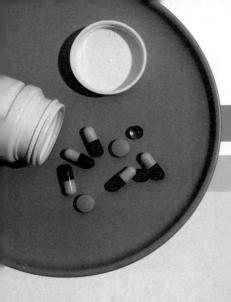

Chapter 8

Medical Ethics

Learning Objectives

- to master some basic skills to build medical words with affixes concerning medical ethics and to expand accurate usage of amphibious words in both general and medical contexts;

- to improve comprehensive linguistic abilities to discuss topics concerning medical ethics;

- to provoke thinking of medical ethics and foster a right attitude towards the issue.

Part 1 Pre-reading Tasks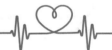

Task 1 Compare and Contrast

*Directions: In medical English, **amphibious words**, a term derived from amphibious animals such as frogs and toads that can live both on land and in water, have flexible meanings in both general contexts and medical contexts. Please consult your dictionaries, write down the Chinese equivalents of the amphibious words in the table below, and pay attention to their different meanings used as **general expressions (GE)** and **medical expressions (ME)** respectively. The first one is exemplified for you to follow.*

Amphibious Words	GE	ME
patient	有耐心的	病人
culture		
discharge		
motor		
pupil		
resident		

(Continued)

Amphibious Words	GE	ME
reproductive		
round		
specialist		
sustain		

Task 2 Read and Translate

Directions: Please read the following 10 pairs of sentences, and keep an eye on the 10 amphibious words you learned from the table in Task 1, which are interpreted differently as GE and ME. Translate the English sentences into Chinese.

1. It worked for me, but it might not work for the less <u>patient</u>. (GE)

    _____

    _____

    He worked in a hospital for ten years nursing cancer <u>patients</u>. (ME)

    _____

    _____

2. We want to expose the kids to as much art and <u>culture</u> as possible. (GE)

    _____

    _____

    To confirm the diagnosis, the hospital laboratory must <u>culture</u> a colony of bacteria. (ME)

    _____

    _____

3. In industry, a worker who is grossly insubordinate is threatened with <u>discharge</u>. (GE)

    _____

    _____

The patients in the control group received routine standard guidance after discharge. (ME)

_____

_____

4. These days it seems we must all submit to the tyranny of the motor car. (GE)

_____

_____

It may induce an inhibitory effect on the sensory nerve and motor nerve, commonly used for sedation and pain relief. (ME)

_____

_____

5. Several pupils were designated as having moderate or severe learning difficulties. (GE)

_____

_____

At night, the pupils dilate to allow in more light. (ME)

_____

_____

6. The building work will go ahead, despite protests from local residents. (GE)

_____

_____

The attending doctor is making a ward-round and discussing the patient's condition with the resident. (ME)

_____

_____

7. The reproductive quality of audio tapes has been improved enormously. (GE)

_____

_____

The research addressed that many young women lacked the knowledge about reproductive health care. (ME)

_____

_____

8. Every good, true, vigorous feeling I had gathered came impulsively round him. (GE)

_____

_____

Making head-nurse quality ward-round is to improve patient satisfaction. (ME)

_____

_____

9. They are each recognized specialists in their respective fields. (GE)

_____

_____

In the first instance your child will be seen by an ear, nose and throat specialist. (ME)

_____

_____

10. Several companies have sustained heavy financial losses due to the unfair competition. (GE)

_____

_____

He sustained an injury to his spine when he fell off his horse. (ME)

_____

_____

Task 3   Lead-in Questions

Directions: Read the questions below and answer them in details.

1. Have you ever heard about medical ethics? What do you think they are concerned about?

   _____

   _____

2. Do you know "placebo effect"? What's your view on it?

   _____

   _____

3. If life can be saved, diseases cured and longevity achieved, what might happen? How will it impact the human world?

   _____

   _____

4. What do you think makes a good doctor?

   _____

   _____

Part 2 Texts

Text A

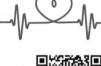

Medical [1]Ethics Education Is Important

1　A 45-year-old man suffered a stroke and is now [2]hospitalized. His **CT scans** reveal a brain [3]hemorrhage. He could die or **fall into a** [4]**coma** for an unknown period of time. Doctors say that though he can be saved, **there are chances that** he may die during the surgery. Even if he lives, he'll probably become disabled. While the doctor believes surgery is the best option, the risks involved cannot be ignored. Here, the doctor is clearly caught **in an** ethical [5]**dilemma**.

2　Medical ethics is a branch of ethics that comprises clinical medicine and related studies. Medical ethics is based on certain values that a medical professional can **refer to** when there are conflicts or confusion. These values are respected for [6]beneficence, [7]non-maleficence, justice and [8]autonomy. Medical ethics is most relevant when professionals have to make a decision of involuntary commitment and treatment.

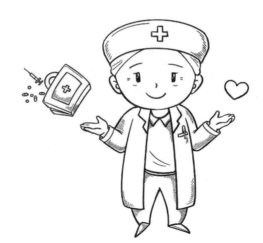

3   Patients or participants may **be exposed to** physical, [9]financial, or psychological risks as a result of the typical Western health care education and research system. To guarantee that students are adequately informed and taught about medical ethics, the basic framework of health care education has to be modified. An ideal medical school is the one that produces proactive physicians rather than reactive ones. The best medical colleges **aim at** [10]inculcating these ethics among their students.

4   Beneficence: The rule of beneficence is the commitment of a doctor to work for the patients based on the various moral standards to ensure and protect the rights of others, [11]forestall hurt, eliminate conditions that will cause hurt, assist people with [12]incapacities, and save people **at risk**.

5   Non-maleficence: It [13]specifies that a procedure must not cause harm to the patient or others in society. [14]Infertility [15]specialists, for example, work **under the assumption that** by pursuing the greater good, they are causing minimal harm. However, as [16]artificial [17]reproductive technologies have low success rates and unpredictable overall outcomes, the patient's emotional condition can be impaired due to this. In such cases, the doctors must consider the risks of harm along with the possible chances of benefit.

6   Justice: Simply expressed, it is the belief that the costs and benefits of [18]innovative or experimental treatments should be shared equally across all social groups. Procedures must follow the spirit of existing laws and be fair to all sides involved. While evaluating justice, the health care professional must consider four primary factors: [19]equitable [20]allocation of restricted resources, conflicting needs, rights and [21]obligations, and potential legal conflicts.

7   Autonomy: One of the primary **guiding principles** of medical ethics is respect for autonomy. Autonomy is all about a person's ability to make their own decisions.

Physicians have a responsibility to create the conditions that allow patients to make their own decisions.

8 In addition, truth-telling and informed ethics do count. One of the most important and well-known processes is truth-telling. You wouldn't want to be around a doctor who keeps secrets about your health and treats you in a secretive manner. Truth-telling is seen as a fundamental moral principle. Hiding information or misleading the patients would be disrespectful of their autonomy. It is very important to have **informed consent** for a medical or surgical operation. Before administering any treatment or therapy, a medical professional must obtain consent from the patient.

9 Medical ethics should be a part of everyday thought, and we need to pay attention to ethical concerns in the health care sector to guarantee that the medical procedures are [22]sound and ethical. The following are the major points that highlight the importance of medical ethics in society. First and foremost, ethical standards promote values that are necessary for effective communication, trust, [23]accountability, **mutual respect**, and equitable medical treatment. Major ethical [24]norms in medical care include informed permission, privacy protection, [25]secrecy, etc. Secondarily, the goal of medical care is to reduce suffering, and ethical norms help in achieving that goal. Last but not least, health care professionals are vital pillars of our modern society, yet there has always been a trust gap between them and the majority of the population for some reason. The recent [26]pandemic has highlighted the fact that a country can only combat health issues if its citizens have the necessary level of trust in the health care system. This trust can be earned when individuals are aware that the health care system follows medical ethics and **is** [27]**intolerant of** any wrongdoings.

10 Every health care professional wishes to be more ethical in their practices, and they want to be sure they're doing the right thing. Ethics helps individuals in making those decisions, allowing them to be more [28]transparent and ethical professionals.

Ravi, J. 2021. What is medical ethics and why is it important? Sooperarticles. Retrieved and adapted on August 15, 2022, from Sooperarticles website.

(768 words)

Notes

1. (Para. 1) Doctors say that though he can be saved, there are chances that he may die during the surgery. 医生说，虽然他可能会被救活，但也可能会在手术中死亡。

2. (Para. 3) To guarantee that students are adequately informed and taught about medical ethics, the basic framework of health care education has to be modified. 为确保学生得到足够的医学伦理知识和教育，我们必须修改医疗保健教育的基本框架。

3. (Para. 4) The rule of beneficence is the commitment of a doctor to work for the patients based on the various moral standards to ensure and protect the rights of others, forestall hurt, eliminate conditions that will cause hurt, assist people with incapacities, and save people at risk. 慈善原则是医生基于多种道德准则做出的服务病人的承诺，承诺会保护他人权益，预防伤害，消除产生伤害的情况，帮助不能自理的人，拯救危险中的人。

   people with incapacities: 残疾人，生活不能自理的人。

4. (Para. 5) It specifies that a procedure must not cause harm to the patient or others in society. 该原则明确指出，治疗手段一定不能对病人或社会上的其他人造成伤害。

   cause harm to：对……造成伤害。

5. (Para. 6) Simply expressed, it is the belief that the costs and benefits of innovative or experimental treatments should be shared equally across all social groups. 简单来说，它代表一种理念：创新性或实验性治疗方法的成本和收益应该由所有社会群体平等分担。

   此句中的 across all social groups 意为"跨越 / 覆盖所有社会群体"。

6. (Para. 9) Medical ethics should be a part of everyday thought, and we need to pay attention to ethical concerns in the health care sector to guarantee that the medical procedures are sound and ethical. 医学伦理应当成为日常思考的一部分，而且我们需要关注医疗保健行业的伦理问题，以保证医疗手段更为健全且合乎伦理。

   此句中的 sound 意为"状况良好的，健全的"。

7. (Para. 9) First and foremost, ethical standards promote values that are necessary for effective communication, trust, accountability, mutual respect, and equitable medical treatment. Major ethical norms in medical care include informed permission, privacy protection, secrecy, etc. 最重要的是，伦理标准提倡的价值观对于实现有效沟通、信任、责任心、互相尊重、医疗平等都是非常必要的。医疗保健的主要伦理规则包括知情许可、隐私保护、保密等。

   informed permission：知情许可。患者具有知情同意权（informed consent），在患者接受医疗的过程中，有权知悉医方对病情的诊断结果及相关资料、拟采取的医疗措施及风险、其他可选择方案等重要内容信息，并可以对医务人员采取的医疗行为做出接受或者拒绝的自主决定权。患者的监护人或代理人具有知情许可时，可以代替病人做出决定。

8. (Para. 9) Last but not least, health care professionals are vital pillars of our modern society, yet there has always been a trust gap between them and the majority of the population for some reason. 最后但仍然重要的一点是，医疗保健专业人士是我们现代社会的重要支柱，但出于某些原因，他们和大多数人之间一直存在信任鸿沟。

trust gap：信任鸿沟，（通常因为双方互相不够了解而产生的）互不信任。

9. (Para. 9) The recent pandemic has highlighted the fact that a country can only combat health issues if its citizens have the necessary level of trust in the health care system. 近期的全球流行病凸显了一个事实：一个国家只有在国民对医疗保健系统具备必要的信任时才能对抗健康问题。

only... if... 意为"某种情况仅在某条件下才能实现"。

Word List

1. **ethics** ['eθɪks] *n.*
   moral principles that govern a person's behavior or the conducting of an activity 道德原则

2. **hospitalize** ['hɑːspɪtəlaɪz] *v.*
   to send sb. to a hospital for treatment 送（某人）入院治疗

3. **hemorrhage** ['hemərɪdʒ] *n.*
   flow of blood from ruptured blood vessels 出血

4. **coma** ['kəʊmə] *n.*
   a state of deep and often prolonged unconsciousness 昏迷

5. **dilemma** [dɪ'lemə] *n.*
   a situation which makes problems, often one in which you have to make a very difficult choice between things of equal importance（进退两难的）困境

6. **beneficence** [bɪ'nefɪs(ə)ns] *n.*
   kindness 慈善

7. **non-maleficence** [ˌnɑːn mə'lefəs(ə)ns] *n.*
   the quality or state of not causing or producing mischief or evil 不伤害

8. **autonomy** [ɔː'tɑːnəmɪ] *n.*
   the ability to act and make decisions without being controlled by anyone else 自主

9. **financial** [faɪˈnænʃ(ə)l] *adj.*

    connected with money and finance 财政的，金融的

10. **inculcate** [ɪnˈkʌlkeɪt] *v.*

    to cause sb. to learn and remember ideas, moral principles, etc., especially by repeating them often 反复灌输，谆谆教诲

11. **forestall** [fɔːrˈstɔːl] *v.*

    to prevent or obstruct (an anticipated event or action) by taking action ahead of time 预先阻止，先发制人

12. **incapacity** [ˌɪnkəˈpæsəti] *n.*

    physical or mental inability to do sth. or manage one's affairs（生理、心理）无能力

13. **specify** [ˈspesɪfaɪ] *v.*

    to state sth., especially by giving an exact measurement, time, exact instructions, etc. 具体说明，明确规定

14. **infertility** [ˌɪnfɜːrˈtɪləti] *n.*

    the state of being unable to produce offspring 不孕症

15. **specialist** [ˈspeʃəlɪst] *n.*

    a doctor who has specialized in a particular area of medicine 专科医生

16. **artificial** [ˌɑːrtɪˈfɪʃ(ə)l] *adj.*

    made or produced by human beings rather than occurring naturally, especially as a copy of sth. natural 人工的，人造的

17. **reproductive** [ˌriːprəˈdʌktɪv] *adj.*

    connected with reproducing babies, young animals or plants 生殖的

18. **innovative** [ˈɪnəveɪtɪv] *adj.*

    introducing or using new ideas, ways of doing sth., etc. 创新的

19. **equitable** [ˈekwɪtəb(ə)l] *adj.*

    fair and reasonable 公平合理的

20. **allocation** [ˌæləˈkeɪʃ(ə)n] *n.*

    the act of giving sth. to sb. for a particular purpose 分配，共享

21. **obligation** [ˌɑːblɪˈɡeɪʃ(ə)n] *n.*

    sth. which you must do because you have promised, because of a law, etc. 义务，责任

22. **sound** [saʊnd] *adj.*

    based on reason, sense, or judgment 明智的，合理的

23. **accountability** [əˌkaʊntəˈbɪlətɪ] *n.*

     responsibility to someone or for some activity 责任心

24. **norm** [nɔːrm] *n.*

     (usually in the plural form) standards of behavior that are typical of or accepted within a particular group or society 规范，准则

25. **secrecy** [ˈsiːkrəsɪ] *n.*

     the fact of making sure that nothing is known about sth. 保密

26. **pandemic** [pænˈdemɪk] *n.*

     a disease that spreads over a whole country or the whole world 传染病，（全国或全球流行的）大流行病

27. **intolerant** [ɪnˈtɑːlərənt] *adj.*

     not willing to accept ideas or ways of behaving that are different from your own 不容忍的，不包容的

28. **transparent** [trænsˈpærənt] *adj.*

     free from pretense or deceit 坦率的

Chunk List

Collocations

1. **in a dilemma** 进退两难

     He was in a dilemma about the party invitation.
     对于是否应邀参加聚会他左右为难。

2. **refer to** 查阅，参考

     You may refer to your notes if you want.
     如果需要，你可以查阅笔记。

3. **be exposed to** 面临，遭受

     They had not been exposed to most diseases common to urban populations.
     他们还未曾遭遇过城市人口常得的大多数疾病。

4. **aim at** 力争做到

     They're aiming at training everybody by the end of the year.
     他们力争做到在年底前人人得到培训。

5. **guiding principle** 指导原则

     His guiding principle has been never to stop learning.
     他的指导原则是永不停止学习。

6. **mutual respect** 相互尊重

     Their marriage was founded on love and mutual respect.

他们的婚姻建立在爱情和互相尊重的基础上。

7. **be intolerant of** 不能容忍

   He was intolerant of both suggestions and criticisms.

   他对建议与批评都不能容忍。

Idiom and Proverb

8. **at risk** 有危险，冒风险

   Hundreds of people are at risk.

   数百人处于危险之中。

(Sub)Technical Chunks

9. **medical ethics** 医德

   Such action was a violation of medical ethics.

   这种行为违背了医学道德。

10. **CT (computed tomography) scan** 计算机层析成像扫描

    Sometimes a CT scan of the abdomen will be necessary.

    有时需要对腹部进行 CT 扫描。

11. **fall into a coma** 陷入昏迷

    The patient had fallen into a coma.

    病人已陷入昏迷状态。

12. **informed consent** 知情同意

    All patients gave informed consent for the treatment.

    所有患者都知情并同意了该项治疗。

Sentence Builders

13. **there are chances that...** 有可能……

    There are always chances that you can get good buys by bargaining.

    你总有机会通过讨价还价买到合算的东西。

14. **under the assumption that...** 假定……

    We are working under the assumption that everyone invited will turn up.

    我们假定每一个受到邀请的人都会出席，并正在进行相应的安排。

Text B

Complex Ethical Decisions

1   UK courts have once again had to ¹**rule on** an incredibly ²fraught case about the

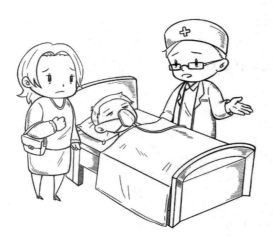

[3]withdrawal of **life support** from a child: 12-year-old Archie Battersbee was found in an unconscious state by his mother and never regained consciousness. The clinical team at Barts Health **NHS** [4]**trust** viewed that it would not be **in Archie's best interests** for him to continue to receive **medical intervention**. Archie's parents disagreed, and sought the court's support to have medical intervention continued. **The court of** [5]**appeal** has ruled that it is legal for the medical team to withdraw his life support, and the [6]**Supreme Court** has **dismissed the family's** final **appeal**.

2   The tragic nature of how Archie became ill and the [7]minutiae of the subsequent legal processes will likely be the subject of public and academic [8]scrutiny for some time. However, what is not **in dispute** is that these decisions are [9]immensely complex, and often include experts considering information that isn't **in the public domain**.

3   Suffering a life-threatening illness or injury may mean that a child requires medical intervention to support basic functions that can maintain life, such as breathing. When they are brought to hospital, clinical teams will **do their** [10]**utmost** to care for and treat a patient if there are any **signs of life**. The professional duties of clinical teams, their ethical standards and the UK legal system all currently include a [11]presumption **in favor of** [12]prolonging life. Beginning an initial [13]**course of treatment** also allows clinical teams time to more fully assess the extent of the patient's illness or injury. Such an evaluation is [14]ongoing as patients differ [15]markedly in terms of the nature and extent of the support they need, and whether and how their body responds to treatment.

4   The questions they would be **looking to** answer include: What is the extent of the patients' illness or injury? How likely are they to recover? If they can recover, what will be their quality of life? If they are unlikely to recover, then what is their current condition? What are the likely benefits and burdens associated with the medical interventions they are currently receiving?

5   Clinical teams also assess what the patients' wishes would be and whether they would have **a preference for** medical intervention being continued or withdrawn.

Adults can make their wishes known through [16]advance [17]directives or lasting **power of** [18]**attorney**. Children, who are legally unable to [19]**avail themselves of** such tools, rely on their parents to make decisions **on their behalf** and to help clinical teams understand what their wishes would be.

6   In cases where there are disputes between families and clinical teams, and the decision is then referred to the courts—as in Archie's case—the ethical question that is often most [20]pertinent is whether medical intervention should continue. In such cases clinical teams either consider the patient to be dead, or they consider continued intervention to be burdensome or harmful to the point that it would be unethical to continue. "Best interest" decisions are some of the hardest decisions that clinical teams are required to make.

7   The [21]likelihood of recovery and the degree of harm an unconscious patient is experiencing can be difficult to **pin down**. These decisions are made more [22]robust by multiple experts, sometimes with a combined experience of a hundred years, who monitor head scans, heart traces, blood tests, [23]pupillary responses and muscle [24]reflexes. They do so repeatedly over days, weeks and even months to establish trends and to understand which of their interventions are helpful and ought to be sustained or increased and which are likely to be harmful and ought to be stopped.

8   In the case of children, in the UK, "best interest" decisions **are** [25]**weighted** even more heavily **towards sustaining life**. As such, a decision to withdraw intervention from a child is likely to rely very heavily on a clinical team's judgment of such intervention being harmful and providing no chance of enabling a life through unsupported means.

9   Recently, ethics committees have had a larger role in supporting clinical teams—they consult families and relevant experts to understand what is **at** [26]**stake** and whether there are aspects of the patient's care that may require further assessment, for example, involvement of additional experts such as a palliative care team.

10   We also need a wider public discussion about what it means to support people artificially through medical means—and to allow children as well as adults to make their wishes known about what they would like to have (and not have) done to them.

Suleman, M. 2022. Complex ethical decisions. Theguardian. Retrieved and adapted on September 4, 2022, from Theguardian website.

(753 words)

Notes

1. (Para. 1) The court of appeal has ruled that it is legal for the medical team to withdraw his life support, and the Supreme Court has dismissed the family's final appeal. 上诉法院裁定，医疗团队撤掉他的生命维持系统是合法的，最高法院驳回了他家人的最终上诉。

2. (Para. 2) However, what is not in dispute is that these decisions are immensely complex, and often include experts considering information that isn't in the public domain. 然而，毫无争议的是，这些决定极其复杂，而且专家们通常会考虑公共视野外的信息。

3. (Para. 3) The professional duties of clinical teams, their ethical standards and the UK legal system all currently include a presumption in favor of prolonging life. 临床诊断小组的专业责任、伦理准则和英国的法律体系目前都包含支持延长（患者）生命的预设。

4. (Para. 5) Clinical teams also assess what the patients' wishes would be and whether they would have a preference for medical intervention being continued or withdrawn. 临床诊断小组也评估患者的愿望，了解他们是愿意继续接受医疗干预还是愿意撤回医疗手段。
   have a preference for：偏好。

5. (Para. 5) Children, who are legally unable to avail themselves of such tools, rely on their parents to make decisions on their behalf and to help clinical teams understand what their wishes would be. 在法律上儿童无法使用这些工具，他们依赖父母代表他们做决定，并帮助临床诊断小组了解他们的愿望。
   on their behalf：代表他们。

6. (Para. 6) In cases where there are disputes between families and clinical teams, and the decision is then referred to the courts—as in Archie's case—the ethical question that is often most pertinent is whether medical intervention should continue. 在家庭和临床诊断小组之间存在争论的情况下，决定权会被移交给法院——就像阿奇的情况一样——与之最相关的伦理问题往往是医疗干预是否应该继续。

7. (Para. 7) The likelihood of recovery and the degree of harm an unconscious patient is experiencing can be difficult to pin down. 神志不清的病人康复的可能性和受到伤害的程度是很难判定的。

8. (Para. 8) As such, a decision to withdraw intervention from a child is likely to rely very heavily on a clinical team's judgment of such intervention being harmful and providing no chance of enabling a life through unsupported means. 在此情

况下，从某个儿童身上撤下干预措施的决定可能在很大程度上依赖临床诊断小组的判断，即这种干预措施是有害的，而且医生也不可能通过无证据支持的（其他）医疗手段使其存活。

9. (Para. 10) We also need a wider public discussion about what it means to support people artificially through medical means—and to allow children as well as adults to make their wishes known about what they would like to have (and not have) done to them. 我们还需要更广泛的公众讨论，去探讨通过人工医疗手段维持人们的生命意味着什么，去探讨允许儿童和成人表达自身意愿，让外界知道他们希望（或不希望）临床医生对他们做什么的意义。

Word List

1. **rule** [ruːl] *v.*
   to give an official decision about sth. 判决，裁定

2. **fraught** [frɔːt] *adj.*
   causing or feeling worry and anxiety（令人）忧虑的

3. **withdrawal** [wɪðˈdrɔːəl] *n.*
   the act of moving or taking sth. away or back 撤走

4. **trust** [trʌst] *n.*
   an organization or a group of people that invests money that is given or lent to it and uses the profits to help a charity 信托机构

5. **appeal** [əˈpiːl] *n.*
   a formal request to a court or to sb. in authority for a judgmentt or a decision to be changed 上诉

6. **supreme** [sʊˈpriːm] *adj.*
   highest in rank or position 最高的

7. **minutia** [mɪˈnuːʃɪə] *n.*
   (*pl.* minutiae) a very small detail 琐事，细节

8. **scrutiny** [ˈskruːtənɪ] *n.*
   careful and thorough examination 仔细检查

9. **immensely** [ɪˈmenslɪ] *adv.*
   very much 非常

10. **utmost** [ˈʌtməʊst] *n.*
    the greatest amount possible 最大可能，极限

11. **presumption** [prɪˈzʌmpʃ(ə)n] *n.*
the act of supposing that sth. is true, although it has not yet been proved or is not certain 假设

12. **prolong** [prəˈlɔːŋ] *v.*
to make sth. last longer 延长

13. **course** [kɔːrs] *n.*
a series of medical treatments, pills, etc. 疗程

14. **ongoing** [ˈɑːŋɡəʊɪŋ] *adj.*
continuing to exist or develop 持续的，仍在进行的

15. **markedly** [ˈmɑːrkɪdlɪ] *adv.*
in a clearly noticeable manner 显著地，明显地

16. **advance** [ædˈvæns] *adj.*
done or given before sth. is going to happen 预先的

17. **directive** [dɪˈrektɪv] *n.*
an official instruction 指示

18. **attorney** [əˈtɜːrnɪ] *n.*
a person who is given the power to act on behalf of another in business or legal matters 代理人

19. **avail** [əˈveɪl] *v.*
to make use of sth., especially an opportunity or offer 利用

20. **pertinent** [ˈpɜːrtɪnənt] *adj.*
appropriate to a particular situation 有关的

21. **likelihood** [ˈlaɪklɪhʊd] *n.*
the chance of sth. happening 可能性

22. **robust** [rəʊˈbʌst] *adj.*
strongly held and forcefully expressed 强有力的

23. **pupillary** [ˈpjʊpɪlərɪ] *adj.*
of or relating to the pupil of the eye 瞳孔的

24. **reflex** [ˈriːfleks] *n.*
an action or a movement of your body that happens naturally in response to sth. and that you cannot control 反射动作

25. **weighted** [ˈweɪtɪd] *adj.*
arranged in such a way that a particular person or thing has an advantage or a disadvantage 有利（或不利）于……的；衡量过的

26. **stake** [steɪk] *n.*

    sth. that you risk losing, especially money, when you try to predict the result of a race, game, etc., or when you are involved in an activity that can succeed or fail

    赌注

Chunk List

Collocations

1. **in one's best interests** 对……最有利

   These reforms were in the best interests of the local government.

   这些改革对地方政府最有利。

2. **in dispute** 有争议

   The cause of the accident was still in dispute.

   事故的原因仍有争议。

3. **in the public domain** 在公共领域；不受版权或专利限制

   This information should be in the public domain.

   这一消息应该为公众所知。

4. **do one's utmost** 尽最大努力

   He did his utmost to persuade me not to go.

   他使尽浑身解数劝我别去。

5. **in favor of** 赞同，支持

   She spoke in favor of the new tax.

   她发表演说，支持新税。

6. **a preference for** 偏爱

   Many people expressed a strong preference for the original plan.

   许多人强烈表示更喜欢原计划。

7. **avail oneself of** 利用

   Guests are encouraged to avail themselves of the full range of hotel facilities.

   旅馆鼓励旅客充分利用各种设施。

8. **on one's behalf** 代表某人

   Mr. Knight cannot be here, so his wife will accept the prize on his behalf.

   奈特先生不能来，因此他的夫人将代他领奖。

9. **pin... down** 确切说明（或理解）

   The cause of the disease is difficult to pin down precisely.

   病因难以解释清楚。

10. **be weighted towards** 有利于

    The proposal is weighted towards smaller businesses.

    这项提议对小型企业有利。

Idioms and Proverbs

11. **look to do** 试图找到做……的方法

    The government is looking to reduce inflation.

    政府正在力求降低通货膨胀。

12. **at stake** 有风险，成败难料

    We cannot afford to take risks when people's lives are at stake.

    人命关天，不容我们冒险。

(Sub)Technical Chunks

13. **rule on** 裁定

    The court will rule on the legality of the action.

    法庭将裁定此举是否合法。

14. **life support** 生命维持系统

    She's critically ill, on life support.

    她病情危急，靠机器来维持生命。

15. **NHS (National Health Service) trust** 国家医疗服务信托

    The NHS trust has mended its ways.

    国家医疗服务信托（机构）已经修正了自己的错误。

16. **medical intervention** 医疗干预

    The honest answer is that no medical intervention is 100% risk free.

    诚实的回答是，没有任何医疗干预是百分之百无风险的。

17. **the court of appeal** 上诉法院

    The case was referred to the court of appeal.

    这个案子被提交到上诉法院。

18. **Supreme Court** 最高法院

    We are awaiting a judgment from the Supreme Court.

    我们正等着最高法院的判决。

19. **dismiss one's appeal** 驳回上诉

    Washington voted to dismiss their appeal.

    （位于）华盛顿（特区的最高法院的大法官们）投票驳回了他们的上诉。

20. **sign of life** 生命迹象

    The body was cold and showed no signs of life.

那躯体冰凉，没有生命迹象。

21. **course of treatment** 疗程

    The course of treatment is long up to two years and the side effects can be severe.

    疗程长达两年，副作用可能很严重。

22. **power of attorney** 代理权；授权书

    The lawyer recommended that Roger give someone financial power of attorney over his affairs.

    律师建议罗杰给某人经济代理权来处理他的事务。

23. **sustain life** 维持生命

    We need food and water in order to sustain life.

    我们需要食物和水来维持生命。

Part 3 Post-reading Exercises

3.1 Read and Answer

3.1.1 Directions: *Read Text A in Part 2 and choose the best answers to the following questions.*

1. What does "dilemma" refer to in the case of the 45-year-old man?

   A. He could not survive the surgery.

   B. He could fall into a coma.

   C. He could be saved by surgery.

   D. He could be saved by surgery but could also die during the surgery.

2. What is/are the significant value(s) in terms of medical ethics?

   A. Beneficence.

   B. Non-maleficence.

   C. Justice and autonomy.

   D. All of the above.

3. What should an ideal medical school do?

   A. It should teach students to avoid medical conflicts.

   B. It should produce proactive physicians rather than reactive ones.

   C. It should make students aware of the ethical dilemma.

   D. It should teach students how to get out of medical confusion.

4. Which of the following is/are NOT mentioned as a primary factor regarding justice?

A. Equitable allocation of restricted resources.

B. Conflicting needs.

C. Rights and interests.

D. Potential legal conflicts.

5. Which is true about medical ethics according to the text?

A. Doctors only need to care about the patients' interest.

B. Medical treatments don't need to follow the existing laws.

C. Patients should be allowed to make their own decisions.

D. Doctors' white lies are allowed for the sake of patients.

6. Why are medical ethics important in society?

A. Because they promote some necessary values.

B. Because they help patients to survive.

C. Because they can comfort citizens.

D. Because they help build the trust gap between doctors and patients.

7. Which of the following does NOT belong to "beneficence" in terms of medical ethics?

A. Protecting the rights of patients.

B. Forecasting hurt.

C. Saving people at risk.

D. Assisting people with incapacities.

8. Which of the following statements is true about "truth-telling" on the part of doctors?

A. Doctors can keep secrets about your health if you have a cancer.

B. Truth-telling is not a basic moral principle.

C. Doctors should inform patients of a medical operation.

D. Hiding information is a legal violation of patients' autonomy.

9. What can be inferred from the text?

A. Medical ethics is only important in the field of clinical medicine.

B. Typical Western health care education is good enough.

C. Medical ethics can solve all conflicts or confusion.

D. Medical ethics involves many aspects.

10. The author mainly tells us _____.

A. what an ethical dilemma is

B. the importance of medical ethics education

C. what the typical Western health care research is

D. how to educate medical students

3.1.2 Directions: *Read Text B in Part 2 and finish the following exercises. Write T for True, F for False, or NG for Not Given in the brackets before the statements based on the instructions below.*

True	*if the statement agrees with the claims of the author;*
False	*if the statement contradicts the claims of the author;*
Not Given	*if it is impossible to say what the author thinks about it.*

(   ) 1. The clinical team thought it would be a great suffering for Archie to continue the medical intervention.

(   ) 2. The court was not on the side of Archie's parents.

(   ) 3. The case about Archie didn't get much attention from the public.

(   ) 4. If a person suffers a life-threatening illness or injury, clinical teams can just withdraw life support according to ethical standards.

(   ) 5. Clinical teams would consider many questions concerning the condition of a patient.

(   ) 6. Parents' decisions on behalf of their children would be assessed by clinical teams.

(   ) 7. Medical intervention has nothing to do with ethics.

(   ) 8. It takes much time and efforts for clinical teams to decide whether to continue or stop medical interventions for an unconscious patient.

(   ) 9. The UK ethics committees would solve all the disputes between patients and their clinical teams concerning the medical interventions.

(   ) 10. Ethics committees won't care about families' opinions.

3.2 Guess and Choose

Directions: *Figure out the meanings of the following medical affixes and choose the best answer from the four choices marked A, B, C and D.*

1. aud, audi (   )

   A. authority   B. autumn   C. automatic   D. hearing

2. pod, podo (   )

   A. foot   B. arm   C. neck   D. breast

3. dent, denti, dento (　　)

    A. density   B. denial   C. tooth   D. dense

4. nas, naso, rhin, rhino (　　)

    A. nasty   B. nose   C. native   D. nature

5. ocul, oculo, ophthalm, ophthalmo (　　)

    A. occasion   B. occurrence   C. eye   D. ocean

6. aur, auri (　　)

    A. auxiliary   B. ear   C. autonomy   D. auction

7. stomat, stomato (　　)

    A. mouth   B. stomach   C. stomachache   D. status

8. gyn, gyne, gyno, gynec (　　)

    A. male   B. gene   C. female   D. gym

9. nephr, nephron, ren, reno (　　)

    A. nephew   B. nerves   C. neat   D. kidney

10. digit (　　)

    A. dignity   B. number   C. code   D. finger or toe

3.3 Read and Think

Directions: Read the following medical words built with the medical affixes from Exercise 3.2 and write down their Chinese equivalents in the table below.

Terminology	Chinese Equivalents	Terminology	Chinese Equivalents
auditory		audible	
pododerm		podocyte	
dentist		dentology	
nasogastric		rhinitis	
oculist		ophthalmology	
aural		auricle	
stomatitis		stomatology	
gynecologist		gynecology	
nephritis		nephroma	
digital		digitus	

3.4 Match and Fill

3.4.1 Directions: Match the medical terms (a–j) in the box below with their definitions (1–10).

a. hemorrhage	b. coma	c. incapacity	d. infertility	e. specialist
f. reproductive	g. pandemic	h. pupillary	i. reflex	j. impair

(   ) **1.** someone's lack of the physical ability to have children

(   ) **2.** excessive discharge of blood from the blood vessels

(   ) **3.** of or relating to the pupil of the eye

(   ) **4.** a disease that spreads over a whole country or the whole world

(   ) **5.** a deep unconscious state, usually lasting a long time and caused by serious illness or injury

(   ) **6.** an action or a movement of your body that happens naturally in response to something and that you cannot control

(   ) **7.** connected with reproducing babies, young animals or plants

(   ) **8.** the state of being too ill/sick to do your work or take care of yourself

(   ) **9.** to damage, weaken or make less good

(   ) **10.** a doctor who has specialized in a particular area of medicine

3.4.2 Directions: Make good use of the medical terms you learned from Exercise 3.4.1 and fill in the blanks in the sentences below. Change the form where necessary.

1. This is a pressing issue because many people are becoming unemployed due to the COVID-19 _____.

2. He was born in November 1940 and died in July 1973 from a mysterious brain _____.

3. Thus, stimulation of one retina will normally invoke _____ constriction in both eyes.

4. Medical _____ have fought a long battle to save his life.

5. A person can be in a(n) _____ for many months before waking up.

6. Extreme stress can _____ the development of the nervous and immune systems.

7. Couples are therefore looking for safer solutions to overcome _____.

8. Almost as a(n) _____ action, I grab my pen as the phone rings.

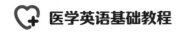

9. The manager has taken sick leave due to his temporary _____ through illness.

10. The _____ system is composed of a series of organs responsible for reproduction of the human race.

3.5 Fill and Translate

3.5.1 Directions: *Choose the correct medical words from the box below to fill in the gaps (1–10) of the passage concerning placebo effect. Change the form where necessary.*

ethical	measurable	clinical	heal	tolerance
minor	physician	placebo	medication	prescribe

Placebo effect, also called nonspecific effect, is the psychological or psycho-physiological improvement attributed to therapy with an inert substance or a simulated (sham) procedure. There is no clear explanation for why some persons experience (1) _____ improvement when given an inert substance for treatment. Research has indicated that the effect may be caused by the person's expectations about the treatment rather than being a direct effect of the treatment itself.

One of the first doctors to deliberately (2) _____ placebos, or inert treatments, was Scottish (3) _____ William Cullen, who mentioned in a lecture series in 1772 having given placebos to patients to appease (安抚) them, not to cure their conditions. Despite Cullen's observations that placebos appeared to produce beneficial effects in some patients, the term placebo effect was not introduced into medicine until the early 20th century.

In modern medicine, (4) _____, including inert drugs and sham procedures, are frequently used in clinical trials that are designed to test new treatments, particularly those developed for neurological and psychiatric conditions. In placebo-controlled trials, enrolled patients are randomly and unknowingly (blindly) assigned to receive either the new medical intervention being tested or a placebo. This prevents patients from knowing what treatment they received, which could cause them to influence study results, and it allows researchers to determine whether the new intervention produces an effect greater than that of the placebo.

The use of placebos in (5) _____ trials has raised important questions in medicine and bioethics. The World Medical Association's (WMA's) *Declaration of Helsinki*, which provides a set of (6) _____ guidelines for medical experimentation on humans, traditionally prohibited the use of placebos in trials when effective therapies or interventions already existed. In 2001, however, the WMA revised its guidelines to allow placebo-controlled trials under certain circumstances, such as when scientific methodology required the use of a placebo or when a new intervention was tested for a relatively (7) _____ health condition.

A significant proportion of new treatments and interventions routinely fail to demonstrate a benefit greater than that of placebos in clinical trials. This has been most notable for certain types of antidepressants and for the application of ultrasound in the (8) _____ of soft tissue injury. In addition, investigations of inert substances have found that the color, the size, and the price of a pill can affect expectations of drug effectiveness. For example, in a report published in 2008, researchers found that test subjects who took an inert substance labeled as a potent pain (9) _____, marketed under a brand name, and sold at a relatively high price experienced greater pain (10) _____ following mild electrical shock to the wrist than people who took an inert substance marketed as a generic pain medication and sold at a comparatively low cost; the brand-name placebo and the generic placebo were the same substance.

3.5.2 Directions: *Translate the underlined sentences from the passage above.*

1. Placebo effect, also called nonspecific effect, is the psychological or psychophysiological improvement attributed to therapy with an inert substance or a simulated (sham) procedure.

2. Despite Cullen's observations that placebos appeared to produce beneficial effects in some patients, the term placebo effect was not introduced into medicine until the early 20th century.

3. In placebo-controlled trials, enrolled patients are randomly and unknowingly (blindly) assigned to receive either the new medical intervention being tested or a placebo.

4. A significant proportion of new treatments and interventions routinely fail to demonstrate a benefit greater than that of placebos in clinical trials.

_____

_____

5. In addition, investigations of inert substances have found that the color, the size, and the price of a pill can affect expectations of drug effectiveness.

_____

_____

3.6 Speak and Write

3.6.1 Directions: *Discuss with your group members and make comments on the phenomena described in Topics 1 and 2 below, and select a representative to report your main ideas to the class.*

Topic 1: cangsheng da yi (苍生大医)

Sun Simiao, a famous physician in the Tang Dynasty (AD 618–907), described an ideal image of a physician as "cangsheng da yi" in his *Essential Formulas for Emergencies*. This term refers to a great physician held in high esteem by everyone and serving all the people. Such a doctor has three basic moral merits: equality, caring and selflessness. Equality requires that a doctor treat all patients with the same care regardless of wealth, social status, or kinship ties; caring demands that a doctor treat all patients with the deepest compassion and empathy; selflessness necessitates treating patients without regard for personal interests. This is the most important component of the concept that "a master physician must have superb skills and sincerity", and the highest manifestation of "the caring heart of a physician", which embodies the humanistic spirit of Chinese medicine.[1]

Topic 2: Hippocrates: The Oath of Medicine (excerpt)[2]

I will prescribe regimens for the good of my patients according to my ability and my judgment and never do harm to anyone.

I will not give a lethal drug to anyone if I am asked, nor will I advise such a plan; and similarly, I will not give a woman a pessary to cause an abortion.

---

1 《中华思想文化术语》编委会 . 2021. 中华思想文化术语·历史卷 . 北京：外语教学与研究出版社，36.

2 Hippocrates. 2002. Greek medicine. *NLM*. Retrieved on July 28, 2022, from NLM website.

But I will preserve the purity of my life and my arts.

I will not cut for stone, even for patients in whom the disease is manifest; I will leave this operation to be performed by practitioners, specialists in this art.

In every house where I come, I will enter only for the good of my patients, keeping myself far from all intentional ill-doing and all seduction and especially from the pleasures of love with women or with men, be they free or slaves.

All that may come to my knowledge in the exercise of my profession or in daily commerce with men, which ought not to be spread abroad, I will keep secret and will never reveal.

If I keep this oath faithfully, may I enjoy my life and practice my art, respected by all men and in all times; but if I swerve from it or violate it, may the reverse be my lot.

3.6.2 Directions: *Discuss with your group members the phenomenon described in Topic 3 below, and write an essay in about 160 words, entitled "To Lie or Not to Lie".*

Topic 3

Imagine that you are a doctor. Now, one of your patients has a terminal illness and is not likely to survive the operation he will undertake. Just as he is about to be anaesthetized (麻醉), he asks you: "Doctor, will I be okay?" Will you tell him the truth or lie to him? A consequentialist (结果论者) ideology supports that lying in this circumstance is acceptable, even though lying itself is not a moral action. If your action has an overall benefit, then the action itself does not matter. In contrast, the deontological (义务论的) approach would suggest that you should not lie to comfort him. That's because according to this theory, lying isn't morally acceptable because it's your obligation not to lie regardless of the consequences. What will you do in this case?

Part 4 Mini-lecture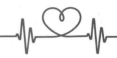

Final Words on Chunks

By the moment you read this lecture, we suppose you've already had some good idea with regard to the definition of chunks, the benefits of learning chunks, the categories of chunks and the way we group chunks in a vocabulary notebook. Besides, you may have already memorized dozens of chunks and become aware of how to use them to improve your productive performance. Good job! Congratulations!

In this last mini-lecture that is supposed to conclude all the previous seven, we'd like to raise three questions to you. We hope you will not only answer the questions honestly, but also always bear these three questions in your mind in the future, if you yearn to continuously improve your spoken and written English.

The first question: Do you believe you have a sufficient stock of chunks in your memory? The second question: Are the chunks in your memory organized in a "clean and tidy" manner, or are they scattered here and there? The third question: Are the chunks in your memory close and friendly to you, or do they look cold and distant?

The first question, of course, reminds you whether or not you have made (or will make) a conscious and persistent effort to learn by heart as many chunks as possible. Linguistic research, at home and abroad, indicates that from the perspective of psycholinguistics, there exist two systems in the mind of a second language learner, namely, a rule-based system and an example-based system. While the former is likely to be generative, which means you can produce seemingly endless sentences according to grammar rules, the latter operates on chunks much of the time and helps accelerate the processing speed in real-life communication. Besides, learning chunks increases the learners' confidence and motivation for learning a second language. It helps with both efficiency and expressiveness since the number and variety of the chunks used in a speech always go hand in hand with the impressiveness of that speech. The more the former, the better the latter. Moreover, even most of the creative language is constructed by chunks which can be cut into smaller strings of words or which could only be used as a whole. Therefore, the edges of having a large repertoire of chunks should never be underestimated.

Once learned, the chunks need to be well organized in your memory so that you can have a quick and easy access to them when you want to use them. This is what the second question above is concerned about. Grouping chunks by meaning, as already illustrated in Chapter 7, is a good way of writing chunks into your vocabulary notebook, because each of them deserves a decent and right place. This way, you are likely to have a more lasting memory of them. But, note that this method has one more benefit, namely the ripple effect. Let's still take the "environment chunks" used in the previous mini-lecture to illustrate this viewpoint. Chunks such as "greenhouse effect" "global warming" "rising sea levels" "shrinking habitats" "carbon emissions" "reduce our carbon footprints" "greenhouse effect" "green taxes" "pristine environments" "household wastes" "destruction of the ozone layer" "alternative energy" "piecemeal conservation", when put together under the topic of environment, can automatically activate each other in real-life communication. Imagine you are discussing the issue of greenhouse effect with someone. You may find, to your surprise, chunks located "near or around" the topic under discussion like the "greenhouse-effect-contributing-factor" chunks ("global warming" "rising sea levels" "carbon emissions", etc.) and the "action-taking" chunks ("reduce our carbon footprints" "introduce green taxes", etc.) are spontaneously activated, which paves the way for your quality production afterwards.

While the second question concerns whether you take good care of the many chunks you've come across, the last one checks whether you have the ability to well harness them to your advantage. Often or properly used, the chunks will be familiar to you and the result is that your English will not be as dry as dust. Seldom used, the chunks will gradually become vague and distant. Chunks need to be learned, to be written down, to be memorized, but most importantly, they need to be used. It is through real and continuous use of the chunks that you will reinforce your memory of them, improve your understanding of the contexts appropriate for them, and finally become a big winner of chunk-learning.

Let's finish this series of mini-lectures with a chunk: "No pain, no gain." Wish you success!